T0323226

TRANSITION to REGISTERED PRACTICE

CHRIS THURSTON & NICK WRYCRAFT

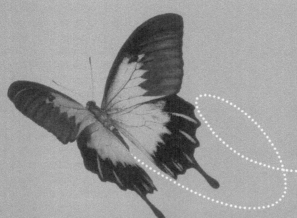

TRANSITION to REGISTERED PRACTICE

from STUDENT to ☆ QUALIFIED NURSE ☆

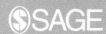
SAGE

Los Angeles | London | New Delhi
Singapore | Washington DC | Melbourne

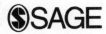

Los Angeles | London | New Delhi
Singapore | Washington DC | Melbourne

SAGE Publications Ltd
1 Oliver's Yard
55 City Road
London EC1Y 1SP

SAGE Publications Inc.
2455 Teller Road
Thousand Oaks, California 91320

SAGE Publications India Pvt Ltd
B 1/I 1 Mohan Cooperative Industrial Area
Mathura Road
New Delhi 110 044

SAGE Publications Asia-Pacific Pte Ltd
3 Church Street
#10-04 Samsung Hub
Singapore 049483

Editor: Alex Clabburn
Assistant editor: Jade Grogan
Production editor: Tanya Szwarnowska
Copyeditor: Joanna North
Proofreader: Rosemary Campbell
Marketing manager: George Kimble
Cover design: Wendy Scott
Typeset by: C&M Digitals (P) Ltd, Chennai, India
Printed in the UK

First published 2020

Library of Congress Control Number: 2019943670

British Library Cataloguing in Publication data

A catalogue record for this book is available
from the British Library

ISBN 978-1-4739-7873-7
ISBN 978-1-4739-7874-4 (pbk)

At SAGE we take sustainability seriously. Most of our products are printed in the UK using responsibly sourced
papers and boards. When we print overseas we ensure sustainable papers are used as measured by the PREPS
grading system. We undertake an annual audit to monitor our sustainability.

Contents

Preface

INTRODUCTION

The nature of nursing is progressing in relation to developing further clinical expertise, and skills and competence, to meet the increasing and changing health care needs of the UK population. This book offers an exciting and appropriate format to guide you as a transitioning student, for all fields of nursing, through the process of leaving the third year to transitioning to qualification. This includes discussion on preceptorship and undertaking CPD and lifelong learning, including revalidation. The book is packed with information and key terms; there are interactive exercises, bullet point summaries of complex issues, and guidance.

RATIONALE

This book focuses on the needs of you as a student transitioning through qualification to your new role as a staff nurse, and offers focused insights with flexible boundaries between the generic and field specific components. The book will enhance your experience by focusing and exploring the main issues which challenge you as nurses, as well as the patient and their families, while intervening in clinical practice. The book also offers supportive text for the period after registration relating to objectives, and the nature of assessed outcomes including revalidation.

THE AIM OF THE BOOK

The aim of this book is to prepare you to adapt and meet changing health care needs within continually adjusting working environments. In order to achieve this, the book's approach has considered your needs and recruitment preferences. It is recognised that some student nurses lack confidence in their knowledge and skills to apply to practice and to manage academic expectations. This book considers these challenges, and within each chapter, information is offered to enhance confidence and competence, for you as the newly qualifying nurse. You may bring to the nursing course life skills that are relevant to practice and these may be utilised within the book in order to give a complete picture of you as an individual and unique nurse.

WHO SHOULD USE THIS BOOK?

This book is intended as a core textbook for you as a transitioning nurse student from an undergraduate degree programme in the United Kingdom, and also, as you newly qualify and explore the opportunities available to you on qualification. It is useful to dip into as you explore the requirements for ongoing CPD and revalidation. The ever changing context of nursing and the evolving health services means that as you near the end of your course and after qualifying you will have to develop the capacity to undertake decisions within the context of policy and risk management. You need to understand the context of preceptorship, supervision, and clinical accountability. There is also a further requirement to remain current for revalidation, and this process alongside the NMC code will be integrated throughout the book.

PEDAGOGICAL FEATURES

Learning outcomes are included in all chapters and set the objectives for you when reading the chapter.

Activities give you the opportunity to undertake reflective problem solving related to the chapter topic.

Practice guidelines relate to current and relevant clinical practice.

Acknowledgements

Chris and Nick would like to thank the many students and qualified nurses, and colleagues that we have had the pleasure to work with over the years who inspired us to create this essential transition in nursing text.

Chris would like to thank her husband Andrew, son Luke and daughter-in-law Claire, along with the grandchildren, for their support as she worked through this essential text.

Publisher's acknowledgements

The publisher is grateful to the following people for their insights and feedback during the review process:

Berni Addyman, University of Bradford

Sheila Dunbar, University of Salford

Peter Ellis, Author and Independent Nurse Tutor

Keith Ford, Fatima College of Health Sciences

Lesley Gratrix, University of Hull

Claire Peers, University of Plymouth

Barbra Steele, Edinburgh Napier University

Editors and contributors

EDITORS

Dr Chris Thurston

Following her nursing qualifications, Chris worked on a number of children's units. She has taught at all levels, from undergraduate students to Master's and the supervision of PhDs. Her role in the university developed from nursing lecturer to Director of Learning and Teaching and finally Head of Department. In this role Chris supported staff who teach nursing. Chris was a Trustee for a young people's hospice. She was drawn to the organisation due to her previous experience of working with young people and her research of their experiences transitioning to adult services. Chris has written books and articles on a number of topics such as safeguarding, children's nursing, transition and multi-professional working. Now retired, Chris continues to support friends and family with their studies and is a Trustee for CAB in the town where she lives.

Dr Nick Wrycraft

Nick Wrycraft is a Senior Lecturer in mental health nursing with Anglia Ruskin University. He has worked at the university for a number of years teaching nursing and health care students. Previously he has carried out research into the use of clinical supervision by health care staff in different clinical settings. Nick has written six previous books, as well as contributing chapters to edited texts, and journal articles on the subjects of mental health nursing and cognitive behavioural therapy. Currently he teaches leadership in nursing and research methodology.

CONTRIBUTORS

Marty Chambers

Marty is Director of Studies in the Faculty of Health, Education, Medicine and Social Care at Anglia Ruskin University. Marty is a registered adult nurse with dual professional and education qualifications. Her areas of interest are the professionalisation of nurse education, pre-registration course curriculum and application and maintenance of the academic regulations to all the courses delivered by the faculty.

Zoe Dodd

Zoe qualified as a mental health nurse in 2018 after changing careers in her thirties. Since qualifying she spent nine months working in a high secure hospital before recently moving to liaison psychiatry and street triage. Zoe will be beginning a part-time PhD in September looking at the impact of professional socialisation on the newly qualified nurse

Patricia Macnamara

Patricia is a senior lecturer in the Faculty of Health, Education, Medicine and Social Care at Anglia Ruskin University. Her expertise is around medical law and ethical issues that occur in the health care setting.

Dr Mary Northrop

Mary was a Senior Lecturer at Anglia Ruskin University working with health care students. Her expertise includes medical sociology, social policy and health promotion. Publications include editing a book for Foundation Degrees and contributing to books on risk, communication and mental health care. Now retired, she is a Trustee for St Helena's Hospice in Essex.

PART I

The beginning of the process

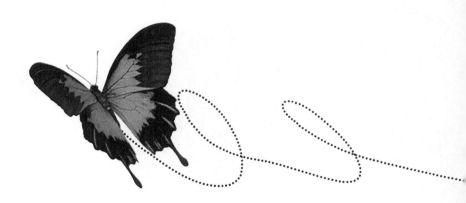

1

The reality of transitioning from student to qualified nurse

Chris Thurston

'The roles of tomorrow's nurses will be even more demanding and special-ised and will require even greater reserves of self-determination and leadership as health care moves into a myriad of settings outside hospital.'

(Willis Commission, 2012)

This chapter will explore the definition of the transitional process and offer expla-nations of your journey from student nurse to a qualified nurse. There will also be a focused exploration of themes related to transition including moral issues and dilemmas, and the need for you to have increased confidence and competence when qualified.

Learning outcomes

- Explore the development of transitional processes in relation to transform-ing from a student nurse to a qualified nurse.
- Critically analyse the professional and moral dilemmas affecting the transi-tion from student to qualified nurse.
- Explore the ways to increase confidence and competence during the transition process.

Making the transition from student to qualified practitioner involves you adjusting to a new and challenging role, accepting additional and different responsibili-ties and being accountable for any actions you undertake. Also, you will need to develop the more complex skills required of a registered nurse. The purpose of transition and then preceptorship is to consolidate the knowledge, skills and attitudes you have already gained in order to demonstrate competence in managing patient care at the point of your professional registration. This chapter will address issues around the need for insight within areas in practice, allowing you to identify the need to maintain and improve the quality of care you offer to patients.

TRANSITIONAL PROGRESSION

Transition can be simply defined as a change for an individual that occurs over time or change in stage of development, or moving from one environment to another, such as school to college, or work (Kralik et al. 2006; Thurston 2010). This fits well with you as a student nurse as you moved through different years of your nursing course to qualification. However, society does not always judge behaviour consistently, and this can lead to you being confused about the responsibilities expected, especially when it comes to making decisions about the health care needs of individuals in your care. Autonomy in nursing practice is often seen as the ideal in nursing, where nurses strive to become successful in gaining clinical independence, leading to a desire to manage your own patients. There are professional challenges such as NMC competency requirements (2018), and socio-legal and ethical issues related to the treatment of patients and accountability from the mentor to you as the student: these are explored in greater detail in other chapters.

It could be argued that there has been an elongation for student nurses gaining responsibility in the current nursing curriculum. Traditionally, first-year students in the early to mid-twentieth century had much more responsibility. Anecdotally from my own experience this was evidenced by first- and second-year students managing wards on night duty and at weekends. This would quite rightly be seen as unsafe practice today. Also, working in parallel there has been a change from School of Nursing training to Higher Education Institute nurse education and from the apprenticeship form of learning to a student-led learning model.

When you scrutinise the transition you are undergoing or have undergone from student to qualification this can be seen from different perspectives, enabling exploration of the ways that you have developed within your professional life. However, there are other factors that you need to include in the patchwork of explanations. These include multiple factors which affect you. It should be acknowledged that any area of your life is influenced by other areas. If you have to take time off your studies because of ill health, it could lead to delay in your course progression but may also affect your clinical skills development. However, a supportive clinical environment will enable you to enhance your management and leadership skills.

Interactions across elements of your professional progress highlight the use of a multi-factorial dynamic approach to transition, which was first discussed in the author's unpublished dissertation, and which is a flexible and realistic model

(Thurston 2010). The influence of factors on your life as a student nurse life is a personal transition, where a change in one area of your life affects all the other areas to a greater or smaller degree. This progressive development occurs for all student nurses but is also a unique experience for you that occurs before and during your student experience and includes personal characteristics including family life and educational ability. Therefore, while a general picture of progression may look similar for all your peers, the specific picture will be shaped by your individual and unique profile.

Therefore, while the concept of transition to staff nurse appears superficially to relate to all your student peers in the third year, it does not seem to be able to explain the transitional experience that some students, including you, may have to progress through during your development into a qualified nurse. Transition is a dynamic process which takes place over time but should not be regarded as a homogeneous progression. Rather than assuming that the ability to achieve academic and clinical competence milestones is the same for all individuals in your student group it is important to recognise that each student's development is unique and individual. A personal transitional profile acknowledges your unique life experience, opportunities and threats that you may experience as an individual due to health, family and the environment. Rather than concentrating solely on educational attainment, there is a need to explore a process that offers explanations for the unique experiences of transition, including factors from a variety of different perspectives.

Rather than being purely a matter of exploring you as an individual passing through your life course, transition is also an active process and there appears to be no consensus as to whether this process has a defined start and finish, or even whether it is linear or cyclical. It can be argued that transitional experience cannot be a purely linear process, but rather is a recurring dynamic multi-factorial process which changes its nature with the realities of the person, both positively for you during periods of wellness or emotional stability and negatively during periods of inadequate professional or family support. Kralik et al. (2006) linked the process to identity and the notion of self and the changes which occur to your personal beliefs because of biographical disruptions; this could include having to move away from home to start your nursing course or qualifying and starting your job as a staff nurse (Thurston 2010).

Transitional definitions acknowledge the changes, rites of passage or maturity of you as a person as you travel from young person into adulthood and regards transition a multi-factorial process which takes your lifestyle, physical attributes, and your family as well as the society you live in and the surrounding environmental influences into account. Much has been made of the growing maturity and increasing empowerment and independence experienced especially during a person's teenage years, and this is true for many students, which may include you as you start a nursing course in your late teenage years. However, there is a variation in the process which includes the progressive nature of a professional course such as nursing with the increasing levels of responsibility required at each stage.

You as an individual have grown physically, socially and psychologically, influenced by all your experiences and relationships; your independence will have increased over time from childhood to adulthood, and change will continue to occur in the passage from being an older adult until death (Robb 2007; Thurston 2010). Levels of independence change, for instance when as a young person you may have started working and living independently. Several factors will now be explored which influence the development of independence and responsibility as a maturing adult and which can be adapted for you as a qualifying nurse. These factors are **Age, Self, Personality, Physical development, Wellness (wellbeing), Intelligence, Environment, Society (neighbourhood), Career (working), Family (home), Finance, Developing relationships, Education,** and **Mobility**, and these elements are commonly cited when talking about transition of any kind (Henderson et al. 2007; Robb 2007; Thurston 2010). They were also part of the focus of the author's PhD dissertation exploring the transition from child to adult (Thurston 2010).

For convenience, the factors are explored separately in the text; however, in reality the factors are interwoven and interrelated. The factors are not just about you as an individual person, such as your physical attributes, but also include other aspects of your life, such as education or the environment and how they have a bearing on your independence, including your chosen career. As you strive to develop into an independent autonomous practitioner, events occur throughout your educational journey which may either accelerate or slow your transitional development; for example, these may include changes in family life, short-term illness or moving to a new house. While some factors may be more significant, such as the death of a partner, or having children, others such as changing job may have less of an impact. The activities below will help you to start to explore your characteristics as a person and indeed as a qualified nurse. As this is a very personal exercise, it seems only right that the author shares her insights as well. Examples used in the text by the author are just that – examples from the author's life. They are not set in stone, and because you are a unique individual you may or may not have had these narratives in your life.

EXPLORATION OF FACTORS

Age

This is a chronological factor, changing from birth to death, and regarding independence it relates to the passage from birth to self-sufficiency as the young person finishes education and starts working (Boyd and Bee 2012; Thurston 2010, 2013). For every person who survives from birth to adulthood, age can be regarded as a chronological and biological measure and is typically seen by society as an indication of increasing competence and independence. However, independence cannot be explored as a purely chronological matter; rather it is the ability and experiences that you as a person negotiate which enhance or reduce your ability to become increasingly independent. Having the opportunity to vote at the age of 18 may be seen by some individuals to make a difference to their lives, while for disaffected young people being able to vote may make no difference to their feelings of alienation and disempowerment.

Therefore, while your age is chronologically determined, it cannot alone determine your ability to behave in a socially approved manner as a young person or adult. While each culture or society decides the age at which a young person can legally vote, have sex or get married, it is you as an individual regardless of chronological age who has or has not the ability to function. As a student nurse you may have come straight from school or college, with very little experience of life outside the home. Perhaps you have had other jobs or caring responsibilities either inside or outside the home. Maybe you have worked in the health care arena for a long time and the nursing course was your approach to consolidating your knowledge and experiences and getting your experiences validated.

Reflect upon your reasons for starting the course at this stage in your life.

Have these reasons changed since you have progressed through different years of the course?

Author's own experience

From an early age I had had caring commitments; I babysat, and cared for my grandmother when needed. I also undertook volunteering in a children's home and a residential school. I finished school and started a pre-nursing course. I was able to study for exams and care for patients in the clinical area with support from the ward staff. This firmed up my commitment to a nursing career. Once I started the nursing course, I realised I got the most satisfaction working with children and families. I finished my general training and followed this with children's nurse training.

Activity 1.1

Self

The second factor which may influence the move from dependence to independence is the notion of self (Aldgate et al. 2006; Thurston 2010). The notion of self is constructed differently depending upon whether a person comes from a collectivist culture or an individualistic society, the latter often seen in the west (www.vocabulary.com). If you come from a collectivist culture you may be less likely to compare yourself with others in terms of personal feelings of self-worth and may be less concerned about your peers being better than you are at skills or activities undertaken. When your feelings of self-esteem and self-worth are constantly optimistic, this enables any experience or challenge to be met in a positive way which further encourages a move towards independence. However, in western society where the individualistic perspective is dominant, a person's view of self can change and fluctuate, depending upon how you are viewed in comparison to peers at school, friends and family. If you grow up believing that you are equal to your peers regarding school activities, there may be positive feelings of self-worth. If you felt inferior due to perceived lack of skills or abilities this may reduce your capability to view yourself in a positive way and may lead to a pattern of lack of self-belief which hinders your ability to develop independence.

Activity 1.2

Think about how you view yourself as a nurse.

How does this compare to how you view your peer group?

Is this reflected in the feedback you receive from your mentors and tutors?

Author's own experience

When I started training to be a nurse, I was often quiet and shy. I got on very well with patients and families but was aware that peers in my group were happier to interact with the multi-professional team. As I grew in competence and confidence, I was able to advocate for the patients, often with the use of diplomacy and humour rather than a more forceful approach. This was reflected in my feedback as a student right up to the present day. I am much happier to have consensus and harmony, than to feel I have had to win an argument.

Personality

The development of your personality occurs within the experiences that take place in the immediate family and the extended social sphere of school or the local community (Thurston 2010). The achievement of an optimistic view of the world, resilience and a supportive social network, may lead you to use opportunities to further broaden your possibilities for personality development. While an individual's personality may have some biological influences from birth in terms of temperament and sociability, these traits are also influenced by the surrounding environment within which you grow (Aldgate et al. 2006; Thurston 2010).

If as a child you had difficulty in mixing with other children but were supported and encouraged by parents and family, you may grow into a person who copes well with strangers. However, if you were aware of your shyness and did not receive support, the awkwardness may reduce your ability to interact with others in society, especially people you do not know, thus reducing your opportunity to develop the skills required for qualification. This view of personality acknowledges both the family and society's view of the person and highlights the uniqueness of you as an individual and your life experiences. Personal experience may enable you to be more assertive in practice or, if the experiences with educational professionals have been disempowering, this could delay your ability to become an independent practitioner.

How well do you handle challenging situations with patients, their families or other colleagues?

Try working on your assertive and communication skills in the clinical setting including dealing with the multi-professional team to perhaps improve these situations.

This should include both active listening and being able to make your view heard.

Activity 1.3

Author's own experience

I have never liked confrontation, I find it stressful and it can lead to poor outcomes for patients if disagreements delay treatment or interventions. I can remember as a newly qualified nurse being with a new house doctor as he tried to site a cannula. I was supportive of the crying child, parent and the doctor, but after the second failed attempt, I calmly told the doctor that they had made enough attempts and that to reduce the continued distress of the child they should get a more senior colleague to help. While the doctor was not pleased, the child and parent were relieved to have the third attempt successfully achieved by a more experienced colleague.

Physical development

Some individuals achieve comparable physical growth and emotional development at roughly the same time, and therefore their minds and emotions and personality are more likely to adjust to the biological changes in similar ways (Boyd and Bee 2012; Thurston 2010, 2013). However, there are wide variations. Some children appear to physically develop in advance of their peers, some at the same time, while others may experience delay in their physical development. Evidence suggests that your physical attributes are a mixture of genetics from your parents, the environment in which you grow, and the level of activity undertaken. If you are someone who had always been above average height, and who likes to undertake physical activities, you could be seen to be older than your chronological age and may be able to develop agility skills which further advance your ability. However, if as a tall child you were seen to act younger and were disciplined according to your perceived age rather than your true age, this

could affect your self-esteem, further restricting your desire to develop physical attributes and delaying the ability to undertake activities with confidence
(Thurston 2013).

Activity 1.4

Write down a few words to describe how you would define yourself
physically.

Have you always been this size and shape?

How has this helped or challenged your role as a student nurse?

Author's own experience

I have always been tall, often one of the tallest in the class at school.
As I was not very agile, I tried to keep to the back of any group activity
that was going on. Being tall has been a great advantage as a nurse:
I could always see above other students' heads if a demonstration or
procedure was occurring. I could carry children around on the ward
quite easily (not to be encouraged as this is clearly not good for your
back or the child). Finally, I was often the same height or taller than
other professionals, which meant not having to look up during eye
contact.

Wellness

When you as an individual are well or have no serious illness, injuries or disabilities throughout life (Kralik et al. 2006; Thurston 2010, 2013), this may lead to an
uneventful progression which reduces barriers or restrictions from society that
impede or cause fluctuations in full independence in older adulthood. An element of this would be your full mobility until old age, having had no restrictions
of movement and adapting to the environment of home and work. Most individuals do not experience life limiting illness, disability or injury until later in life. This
may mean that you have an uneventful life course until you pass middle age,
and then either an accident or illness may affect your level of independence. For
some patients this means an end to independent living and a requirement for
health care and support, from family and/or health professionals.

   For others, determination of spirit and appropriate practical support and services may mean that while they require input at times for their illness on their own
terms, they maintain a level of independence within the context of the illness or
disability (Law Commission 2008). Where this is the case, illness transition will
have varying influences on you and on other individuals, which may become
a significant factor as you age, and influence the level of independence which
may supersede the optimal level of independence during late adulthood. This
chronological sequence of events is an assumption which, while holding true

for some, varies when you have the knowledge that any feelings of physical wellbeing and illness may be transient and may become progressive or less frequent as you reach older adulthood.

Did you develop or were you born with any long-term conditions?

How has this affected you nursing career?

Does this make a difference to how you relate to patients and families?

Author's own experience

I have been very fortunate growing up not to have any long-term illness or medical conditions; however as I got older long-term conditions have occurred. I have also broken a few bones and therefore at times have been restricted in my mobility. This has enabled me to gain some insight into the challenges of using a wheelchair or crutches, when having to carry on with the activities of everyday living.

Activity 1.5

Intelligence

Success in preordained intelligence tests can be achieved if you have no cognitive disabilities that restrict aptitude to new knowledge and skills learnt (Aldgate et al. 2006; Boyd and Bee 2012; Thurston 2010, 2013). Independence is enhanced if you can utilise your innate intelligence and learn to solve problems with support from family, school and your social network and develop skills as you transition into adulthood. However, if you were not encouraged to work through problems with support, but were always offered the solution, it may delay your ability to be independent. While the use of intelligence tests has some value, it does not readily acknowledge your individual life experiences and opportunities which occur outside the remit of innate abilities. There also needs to be acknowledgement that IQ tests are devised in certain ways, and that some children and young people may perform poorly on such tests which fail to take into account their knowledge, abilities, gender or culture. However, these children may still perform challenging tasks in other environments; for example a child who has not had the opportunity to learn to read and write may have the ability to repair intricate machinery or offer complex care to another individual (Berk 2012). As a student nurse you were required to gain qualifications to start the course and were expected to pass exams and demonstrate competencies throughout the course. The ability to undertake these problem-solving exercises has shown your knowledge and intelligence. Others will not have known how hard or easy you found the process, however. Some of your peers may appear to have sailed through their exams with very little study or work while others may have had to work very hard to achieve a similar result.

Has study been a challenge or an enjoyment for you as a child or young person?

Critically reflect on how you prepare for an exam or assignment.

Do you study and prepare from the beginning or you a last minute person?

Do you seek out support or try to work things out by yourself?

Author's own experience

Study for me was always a challenge. I enjoyed finding out the information and gaining knowledge. I found it much harder to express this in written words. Throughout my education, from school, college, nursing and university, I redrafted my work many times. This, however, is no reflection on my intelligence but rather my challenges with writing due to dyslexia. As I progressed through my career, I have accepted that I must work harder than others to achieve the same result. This also made me stronger as it has helped me develop strategies to make the process less challenging. This barrier to success has not stopped me, rather it has spurred me on to work on my strengths in practice.

Environment

If you have lived in a safe environment and been able to attend school or work in an atmosphere which is conducive to healthy living you are more likely to thrive (Boylan and Dalrymple 2009; Robb 2007; Thurston 2010). Moving to a new house specially to start your nursing course may be an enjoyable process, as you could finally have your own room and private space. You may on the other hand have had a house move which caused challenges due to the loss of a network of friends and peers from school or you may have had to acclimatise to a different environment, which might include unfamiliar living conditions and reduced space. The environment plays a significant part in the development of everyone and this is reflected in your life experience of studying nursing; it is important to develop different resilience strategies depending upon the support you receive from family, friends, course peers, tutors and supervisors or mentors in practice.

How frequently did you move around as you were growing up?

Did you stay at home or move to accommodation when you started the nursing course?

Reflect upon what it is like to move from one clinical environment to another clinical environment.

Author's own experience

I was very fortunate to live in the same house growing up, until I started nursing. And I also had the same accommodation during most of the course. The area I found most challenging was going from clinical area to clinical area. Each new placement was for me like a new country. I felt I had to learn new words about medical conditions and medications, and also investigations and treatments. Finally, I had to develop relationships with new members of nursing and medical staff. This left a deep impression on me. I can still remember the nurses who were patient and spent time with me, even though they were busy. I tried to incorporate this into my support for students on the wards and at university.

Society

Society can either be viewed as supportive of diversity and the unique needs of different groups or individuals, or alternatively as placing restrictions or barriers in the way, due to assumptions about cultural beliefs and values (Holdsworth and Morgan 2005; Thurston 2013). You may live in a community which enhances health and wellbeing with community networking, mutual support and acknowledgement of personal values and beliefs. You may live in a community which offers some opportunities for shared values but which also resorts to assumptions and discrimination when a person is viewed as different because of culture, disability or sexuality. This can lead to disempowerment and restriction of movement and independence if you felt frightened or ashamed to leave the house (Thurston 2010, 2013). The social attitudes that others display towards you if you are different from most of the population in a community, neighbourhood or society can lead to further discrimination and prejudice. If you decided to become a nurse and that was not seen as a typical profession for someone in your family or community because of gender, sexuality or perceived lack of status, it can make it much harder to ask for support or further guidance from close family and the local community.

How did your family and friends and the local community react to you starting the nursing course?

As you are completing your education and transitioning to qualified nurse has this changed?

Will the experiences you have shared with family and friends help to change their view on the professional status of nursing?

Activity 1.8

(Continued)

(Continued)

Author's own experience

Nursing was an appropriate career for the women in our family: I and two of my siblings qualified as nurses, while another two siblings under-took caring roles. Both my parents expressed how proud they were of my achievements. My dad was extremely proud when I undertook my children's course at Great Ormond Street. I went on to undertake further study and this was a chance to show to family and friends that nursing was both academic as well as competency based.

Career

To obtain the career of your choice when transitioning into adulthood you have had to develop the skills and physical abilities to begin to function and work with or without your parents' support, towards a career through school, college or university and gaining the qualifications required (Kehily 2007; Thurston 2010). This process occurs for most people; however, the time taken varies from person to person, and is also dependent upon when you decided on your career. If you went to college before university your progression to full independence may be longer than if you were 16 years old when you started work, and for some the opportunity to pursue your chosen career may materialise late due to illness, disability or deprivation (Henderson et al. 2007). You may have taken longer to gain the necessary qualification to begin the course, had a different career before deciding on nursing, or you may have had your family first. All these experiences will have an impact on you as you start the course and the life skills you have already gained that you are able to bring to the course.

Activity 1.9

Was nursing your first choice of career?

If it was not, what did you do first?

What experiences changed your mind?

As you are coming to the end of the course, are you planning on where you want to work?

Are you aware of any further study or competencies you require?

Author's own experience

As I mentioned, nursing was my chosen career from quite early on. However, as I went through the course, I began to see the different paths I could take. There was no clinical area I did not like. However, when I went to the children's ward, it felt like my professional and clinical home. The relationship with nursing and medical colleagues alongside the partnership working with children, young people and their families felt right. I discovered a level of honesty and commitment from the multi-professional team that I personally had not experienced elsewhere.

Family

The family is often cited as a significant factor in both social and personal developmental progression and is significant for everyone. How family is defined has changed over time within western society, from a married couple with children to individuals who may live together in households.

Despite some weakening of bonds, personal intimate relationships, such as with parents, siblings and grandparents, continue to be an important source of support, care and identity. Some aspects of motherhood and fatherhood may be changing, but parenting is still crucial for nurturing children, whether that be in single parent households, post-divorce parenting or gay and lesbian partnerships.

(Harden et al. 2013)

If as a child you had a family where warmth, practical help and emotional support were present this may enable you to have the stability and structure to move steadily and progressively through the transition from youth to adulthood and increasing independence. However, dynamics within families can vary over time, for example this could occur when siblings are born, or parents separate (Holdsworth and Morgan 2005; Kehily 2007; Thurston 2010). Therefore, your experience as a family member may be different to that of your siblings or cousins, or younger relatives, and may affect how you cope with other intimate relationships as an adult or nurse and with your own family.

Where do you come in your family?

Is the family small or large?

Are there more boys than girls?

Do you see other relatives often?

How do you think your family relationships have enabled your ability to make professional relationships?

Activity 1.10

(Continued)

(Continued)

Author's own experience

I come from a large family, both of siblings and cousins. This enabled me to learn to get on with other people and try to resolve issues. As I said earlier, I do not like conflict and this was a challenge as I found it difficult to speak up at the beginning of the course. Once I had had a child I could more easily empathise with parents when their children were ill. This can be both a strength and a challenge as parents do not want to see a professional being overcome with grief when their child is seriously ill. My professional relationship with child patients and their families was to show my emotions and to befriend them during their illness journey. I was however clear that I was not their friend as I was there to support them.

Finance

Financial issues are a factor often explored as an influence on development, and how parents or guardians handle these responsibilities and whether individuals have their needs for clothes, food, warmth and educational and social activities met. Family resources and incomes are challenged by a multitude of elements including parental education, lifestyle choices, disability, and social class and deprivation, while the dynamic within the family can change and become less supportive of you as the child, or young person or young adult (Holdsworth and Morgan 2005; Thurston 2010). However, the quantity of money that comes into the home does not guarantee a happy or healthy life for the family; rather it is the way resources are used which may be significant (Walker and Thurston 2006, and Thurston 2010).

Activity 1.11

Were you aware of the finances in your home as you were growing up?

Did money play a part in the timing of starting the course?

Have finances been challenging during the course?

What steps have you had to take to balance resources with studying?

Author's own experience

I had several part-time jobs before I started nursing, and I was fortunate that during my nursing course I received a salary. Once I qualified some of the courses I undertook were paid for and others were self-funded.

This meant I had to juggle work with study and child care. While I found this very hard at times, looking back it was the support of my husband, friends and colleagues at work which made this a success.

Developing relationships

As you progressed through your childhood with or without the support of family and the involvement of friends you became young adults and therefore more independent (Kehily 2007; Robb 2007; Thurston 2010). Your social network of friends in childhood whether during school or leisure activities encourages the development of communication skills that are beneficial when transitioning to college or work and beginning adult relationships. You may have developed and kept friendships throughout your life, some starting in childhood, or you may find friends during the transition through school, college or career (Kehily 2007). Friendships can be positive and enhance self-worth and communication skills, or alternatively your relationships could have been challenging as you tried to conform to the peer group, even when this may have led to physical or emotional self-harm (Barham 2004). This could be significant for you if your peer group growing up did not want to study or pursued risk-taking behaviours.

How many friends have you still got from childhood?

How many friends have you had for over five years?

How many friends have you made since you have been on the course?

Do you think you will stay in touch with these friends after you finish the course?

Activity 1.12

Author's own experience

I have had a handful of friends that I have known for a very long time. These friends are from college, nursing, as past neighbours and at university; some I met over three decades ago. My closest friend and I started our nursing course together and have been with each other through health, illness and the birth of children. I believe that you cannot choose your family, but you can choose your friends. I have had fleeting friends who have been in my life for a short time. My great support has been from my close network of friends, especially those who know what it means to be a nurse or carer.

Education

Education can be life enhancing, giving you opportunities for developing skills which would be beneficial to the transition through school, college and on to work. A good educational experience may enable you to undertake studies to pursue and enter the career of your choice (Robb 2007; Thurston 2010). However, if your school experience was a challenge from lack of resources or practical support, you may have had barriers which restrict qualifications or career choice (Thurston 2010, 2013). If you have had learning needs, or survived bullying or other experiences or conditions which affected your learning experience, this may have made school a difficult place to be.

Activity 1.13

Did you enjoy school?

Has this affected how you have experienced the nursing course?

What strategies have you put in place to support you when you are struggling on the course or with studying?

Author's own experience

I remember having learning needs from early in my school experience. I did not understand the issues and often I was just seen as lazy or slow. At that time there was no specific professional who offered support and it was only through the kindness of a wonderful teacher, Miss Adams, in my final year of junior school that I got the support I needed to catch up with my peers. Studying for A levels and then the nursing exams was difficult for me. I was supported by a dedicated nurse tutor, Ms Goslin, who went above and beyond to help me achieve success in my state finals exam. These positive experiences went alongside a significant number of negative experiences. I learnt how not to treat people from my negative learning experiences and to become more assertive when asking for support, and I gained respect for professionals who place patients and/or students at the centre of their working lives.

Mobility

As you grow, you start with physical mobility, learning to walk and then cycle, along with social mobility skills such as learning how to catch a bus, and becoming more socially active by undertaking activities with peers and friends or during career progression (Henderson et al. 2007; Montgomery 2007; Thurston 2010). You may pass a driving test and finally become independent enough to leave home, for college or your own accommodation or independent travel. People learn these skills at different rates. Montgomery (2007) discusses moving (mobility) in broad terms related to increasing independence and decision making for the young person. She goes on to remark that moving for some may be transformational in terms of exploring other countries or cultures and a point of transition from the culture of youth into that of young adult. However, moving may also be about crisis and disruption, as the environment may be riskier. Starting the nursing course may have raised a few dilemmas for you, such as: Where should you go to study? What field or branch of nursing do you want to pursue? Do you want to do the course full-time or part-time and what will this mean for you and your family?

Why did you choose the course you did?

Why did you choose the location?

Will you stay at the same hospital when you have finished the course?

If not, why not?

Activity 1.14

Author's own experience

I decided to move away from home but not too far, staying in the same county. This enabled me to have some independence, but I was also able to get home quickly if I needed to. I did not return home as I started a job close to the hospital where I undertook my course. This worked well for me as I was still in the same county as my family home, but I also got to know a different part of the region. I then moved again a couple of years later to the clinical area where I remained until I went to teach children's nursing at the university.

The factors explored in this chapter are not a definitive list but rather a reflection of some of the factors included in approaches that help to define and explore your experiences of being a student nurse transitioning to qualification. This acknowledges the intimate relationship between transition into qualification and professional independence. The chapter shows the relationship between multiple factors and independence and transition to qualification, and this has led to an acknowledgement of the interactive relationship of the factors discussed and how they all play a part in your professional growth.

THE TRANSITION FROM STUDENT NURSE TO QUALIFIED NURSE

The transition from student nurse to qualified nurse discussed here offers a challenge to the view of a longitudinal progression through your nursing course, and to the view that your process of transitioning into a qualified nurse will be the same as that of your peer group of students, occurring in the same time span and with similar experiences. Adopting a restrictive approach detracts from you and every other student nurse, and your and their unique life experiences which led to the decision to become a nurse, whether influenced by culture, gender, class, health experiences or family.

The nursing course may lead to changes in your psychological and intellectual ability, competency and confidence, and can be seen to run parallel to the transition into adulthood as in the beginning of the course you start as a novice student nurse and become more competent as you progress through the course, thus enabling you to take on more responsibility and requiring less supervision. There will be changes in your socio-cultural standing, especially when as a student nurse you transition into the third year and are seen as a senior student, in both the clinical setting and in the university. This leads to changes in your circumstances or situation, such as learning how to give more complex medication or handle more complex dressings, through to managing a group of patients with support from colleagues and junior staff (Kralik et al. 2006; Thurston 2013).

Activity 1.15

What knowledge and skills were you expecting to gain during the final year of the course?

In management?

Working with the multi-professional team?

Did this occur?

A qualitative study of nursing student experiences of clinical practice by Sharif and Masoumi (2005) concluded that 'nursing students experienced anxiety as a result of feeling incompetent and lack of professional nursing skills and knowledge to take care of various patients in the clinical setting'. While this was over a decade ago, some students still express these concerns when progressing through the nursing course. Steivy et al.'s (2015) study explored with a small number of student nurses their experiences of learning in clinical areas using focus groups and interviews. They concluded that:

> integration of both theory and practice and opportunities for application and laboratory skills enable student nurses to learn effectively, to feel confident with their skills, and to become competent in taking care of patients.

(Steivy et al. 2015)

As a student who has successfully made the transition to the third year and then as you qualify, you will have drawn upon experience both in the clinical area supported by your mentors and in the Higher Education Institution (HEI) with your personal tutors.

Abstract 1.1

'Research notes (student nurses' views) final-year student nurses' perceptions of role transition'

Doody et al. (2012) *British Journal of Nursing*, 21(11), Abstract

Role transition can be both challenging and exciting. This study presents the findings of phase one of a two-part study conducted by Deasy in 2011, which explored final-year student nurses' (n =116) perceptions and expectations of role transition. The students were registered on four-year BSc nursing programmes at an Irish university. Data was analyzed using SPSS. A response rate of 84% was achieved. Over half of respondents said they were adequately prepared for the post of registered nurse. Respondents generally perceived themselves to be competent across a range of domains: managing workloads; prioritizing care delivery; interpersonal skills; time management skills; ethical decision making; and providing health information and education. In contrast, not all were confident about their knowledge and many expected the transition to be problematic. Most expected to be supported and to receive constructive feedback. Recommendations include nurturing supportive work environments to reduce stress and increase confidence.

Doody et al. (2012) highlighted both the development that third-year students in the study have achieved and the concerns they have when they qualify. This study goes on to say that support is required for you and all third-year student nurses not just on qualifying but during the whole transitional process. It is beneficial to NHS staff resources for all students to become part of the independent professional workforce and not to be dependent on others for constant close supervision. However, part of that growing independence is dependent upon the support you receive during transition, especially from being signed off as competent in practice as a student, through the preceptorship process as a newly qualified nurse. If as a student nurse you receive positive and constructive mentorship or support from coaches, this will enable you to continue both your personal and professional development into the new area of qualification. Moving this forward will also enable you to support junior colleagues including students earlier on in their course.

Activity 1.16

List the responsibilities that become more relevant to you as you gain more responsibility during the transition from the course to qualification.

How may this be different if you as the student are studying for a different part of the register?

An area closely related to increasing responsibility is advocacy and how as student nurses during your course you viewed the support you can offer to patients, clients and their families when they require interventions, either for social or physical needs. Mentors or supervisors as you progressed through each year of your course may have offered a developmental approach to you when working in partnership with patients and families. This approach can often be seen as generic and chronologically based, fitting you into already defined developmental stages of the nursing course rather than acknowledging the unique features of you as a student nurse and your strengths and personal experience working in the clinical or community setting. Good supervisors will clearly have gone above and beyond this, but when the clinical environment is busy this may not have occurred.

For you as a student this adjustment to a variety of environments can highlight further concerns, especially juggling study and home and placements (Thurston 2013; Valentine and Lowes 2007). The experience of acquiring the skills to adapt and survive in clinical placements is difficult as cultural normalities around language, behaviour and lifestyle seem to shift more quickly than some nursing students can often comprehend or adjust to (Henderson et al. 2007; Thurston 2013).

The elongation of preparation for nursing practice can be seen in the extension of time in the skills labs and in the HEI before clinical practice to encourage students to marry theories of nursing to practical applications in the clinical setting. It could also be a means of preparing you the student for the stress involved in the clinical environment. During transition to qualification you may, with positive experiences in study and clinical practice, advance your level of self-worth and identity as an individual. This may have been a consistent feature of your psychological development to the present time, alongside developing further your own personal beliefs and values. While many of the skills and competencies may seem of value to student nurses, especially in terms of increasing abilities to problem solve and have insight into how your caring behaviour may, affect the patients' health and safety, there has to be some critique of completion of these skills in relation to the theory/practice, gap. Considering the social perspectives of nursing, focusing on the dynamics of interaction between you and your immediate environment, you may be influenced by the environment you are in, including your relationships with peers and superiors, and the experience of transition through to qualification.

During the transition to qualified nurse, you may have many positive clinical experiences advancing feelings around self-worth and identity as a nurse, alongside developing further personal and professional beliefs and values especially around the '6Cs' date and NHS values (2015). While many of the nursing tasks are of value to you as a student nurse, especially in terms of increasing abilities to problem solve and have insight into patient health and wellbeing, when you encounter situations or individuals who have a negative affect on your progression this can stem progress and, on some occasions, lead students to leave the course.

Because individuals learn through their environment, you may be aware of the changes in patients' physical and mental health and can recognise that wellness and illness can exist at the same time (Glasper and Richardson 2010; Thurston 2013). However, most individual patients consider health to be achievable by taking care of oneself and are aware of the internal clues to health including their own role in promoting their own health. While some patients can be compliant with their treatment regime, this does not preclude others from being noncompliant, especially if the person has a long-term medical condition involving further admissions to hospital. Therefore, you may develop a more cynical approach to health and wellbeing, which acknowledges the lack of consistency regarding maintaining health.

As an individual you may feel different to your peers both in terms of confidence and knowledge and characteristics. This awareness of personal difference is not always considered in general educational theories regarding professional development as the assumption is usually made that individuals who are student nurses will be able to keep pace with the commitment of the course, regardless of caring commitments or financial constraints. As you work through this book, take your own pace. There will be activities which really help and others which do not resonate with your narrative. Use your professional and personal judgement to decide what areas you need to work on and the areas which can be explored later.

REFERENCES

6Cs and NHS values, 2015, www.hee.nhs.uk/about/our-values; 6 Cs 2016, www.england.nhs.uk/leadingchange/about/the-6cs, accessed June 2019

Aldgate, J., Jones, D., Rose, W. and Jeffery, C. (eds) (2006). *The Developing World of the Child*. London: Jessica Kingsley.

Barham, N. (2004). *Disconnected: Why Our Kids Are Turning Their Backs on Everything We Thought We Knew*. London: Random House.

Berk, L.E. (2012). *Child Development*, 9th ed. Boston: Pearson.

Boyd, D. and Bee, H. (2012). *The Developing Child*, 13th ed. Harlow: Pearson Education.

Boylan, J. and Dalrymple, J. (2009). *Understanding Advocacy for Children and Young People*. Maidenhead: Open University/McGraw-Hill.

Doody, O., Tuohy, D. and Deasy, C. (2012). Final-year student nurses' perceptions of role transition. *British Journal of Nursing*, 21(11): 684–8.

Glasper, A. and Richardson, J. (eds) (2010). *A Textbook of Children's and Young People's Nursing*, 2nd ed. Edinburgh: Churchill Livingstone.

Harden, J., Marsh, I., Keating, M. (2013). *Sociology: Making Sense of Society*, 5th ed. Harlow: Pearson Education.

Henderson, S., Holland, J., McGrellis, S., Sharpe, S. and Thomson, R. (2007). *Inventing Adulthoods: A Biographical Approach to Youth Transitions*. London: Sage.

Holdsworth, C. and Morgan, D. (2005). *Transitions in Context: Leaving Home, Independence and Adulthood*. Maidenhead: McGraw Hill Education, Open University Press.

Kehily, M.J. (ed.) (2007). *Understanding Youth: Perspectives, Identities and Practices*. London: Sage/Open University.

Kralik, D., Visentin, K. and Van Loon, A. (2006). Transition: a literature review. *JAN: Journal of Advanced Nursing*, 55(3): 320–9.

Law Commission (November 2008). *Adult Social Care: A Scoping Report*. London: The Law Commission.

Marsh, I. (2013). *Sociology: Making Sense of Society*, 2nd ed. Harlow: Pearson Longman.

Montgomery, H. (2007). Chapter 2: A comparative perspective; and Chapter 9: Moving. In M.J. Kehily (ed.), *Understanding Youth: Perspectives, Identities and Practices*. London: Sage/Open University, pp. 45–72 and 283–312.

Nursing and Midwifery Council (NMC) (2018). *Ensuring public safety, enabling professionalism*. www.nmc.org.uk/concerns-nurses-midwives/fitness-to-practise-a-new-approach/

Robb, M. (ed.) (2007). *Youth in Context: Frameworks, Settings and Encounters*. London: Sage/Open University.

Sharif, F. and Masoumi, S. (2005). A qualitative study of nursing student experiences of clinical practice. *BMC Nursing*, 4: 6.

Steivy et al. (2015). Final-year student nurses' perceptions of role transition. *British Journal of Nursing*, 21(11): 684–8.

Thurston, C. (2010). The life and transitional experiences of eight young people with cystic fibrosis (CF). A thesis in partial fulfilment of the requirement of Anglia Ruskin University for the degree of PhD in Social Science.

Thurston, C. (ed.) (2013). *Essential Nursing Care for Children and Young People: Theory, Policy and Practice*. London: Routledge.

Valentine, F. and Lowes, L. (eds) (2007). *Nursing Care of Children and Young People with Chronic Illness*. Oxford: Blackwell Publishing.

Vocabulary.com. www.vocabulary.com/dictionary/collectivist, accessed January 2019.

Walker, S. and Thurston, C. (2006). *Safeguarding Children and Young People – A Guide to Integrated Practice*. Dorset: Russell House Publishing.

Willis Commission (2012). Raising the Bar, Shape of Caring: A Review of the Future Education and Training of Registered Nurses and Care Assistants. Lord Willis, Independent Chair – Shape of Caring Review Health Education England.

2

Preparing for your first job
Nick Wrycraft

The philosopher Lao Tzu said that

> *'A journey of a thousand miles begins with the first step.'*

But as anyone who has travelled knows, the journey begins even before that point as we prepare and consider what we will need along the way. Yet, as is the case with many journeys, we cannot always anticipate what we will need, while what we might think will come in handy turns out to be of no use at all. In this chapter we discuss the extent to which you can plan and prepare to apply for your first job.

This chapter explores finding a job and deciding where you may want to work both in terms of location, and in terms of type of nursing and age group. It will explore how to analyse job details and supporting materials from the employer. The chapter will discuss the development of CVs and preparation for interviews, including potential questions, and the extent to which you can plan and prepare to apply for your first job.

Learning outcomes

- Understand the job application and screening process.
- Identify what should be included in a CV.
- Consider how to structure a personal statement and know what to include.
- Understand how to prepare for the interview.
- Have thoughts about how you might feel about the outcome.

Perhaps the most important factor of all in looking for, finding and preparing to apply for a job is our attitude, and the mind-set that we have when we begin the journey. Accepting that we will be somewhere that we do not know, surrounded by new possibilities is exciting but also daunting. Being open and receptive to this experience will help us gain as much as we can and at the same time mean we can adapt and learn quickly. This chapter is written from the perspective that change is something for which we can make well-judged practical preparations, and rather than regarding it with fear and apprehension we will fare better by regarding the challenge as an exciting learning opportunity through which we can develop.

Your first qualified nursing job represents a milestone in your life and career. In hindsight it will assume great significance whatever you then go on to do. Yet the process of finding this post is very similar to seeking any other job. It is worth reflecting on just how far you have come, and to devise a good plan in order to find a job that suits your personality, skill set and new identity as a registered nurse. After so much time spent studying and training, working as a qualified nurse can feel as though you are beginning nursing for real. This has the potential to be stressful and place you under significant pressure. Therefore, it is important to choose a job where the transition from senior student to qualified and competent staff nurse will be well-managed (see **Chapters 2 and 3**), and where you will receive the level of support and feedback that is necessary to help you feel confident in making this change and help reduce the inevitable stress.

In this chapter we will look at preparing for your first job as a qualified nurse. There are a number of practical issues which need to be thought about. Choosing which jobs to apply for is vital, as it is necessary to think about what the role entails but also whether you are suited in terms of your preferences, skills and capabilities.

Below we discuss how to decide on jobs to apply for, and putting together an application, including the importance of the job specification and the function of essential and desirable characteristics. The chapter then progresses to look at researching the role, compiling a CV before writing the personal statement, how to prepare for the interview, and then what to do after the interview.

CHOOSING A JOB

When considering applying for your first qualified nursing job there can be a dilemma. It is tempting to apply for numerous posts to increase your chances of being successful. On the other hand, you may prefer a more targeted approach and choose a few specific posts upon which to focus your efforts. Both approaches have advantages and disadvantages which we will consider next.

Jobs are well advertised, with Trusts generally having pages advertising vacancies on their websites, as well as there being specific sites advertising posts, and once you have a CV this can be reused for multiple other applications, while the online process is quite easy, quick to complete and straightforward. Often even the wording of cover letters can easily be adapted to allow for repeated use for different posts. Therefore, applying for numerous jobs is easy to do, and may seem to increase your chances of success, while gaining experience in interview situations will enhance your skills in this area. However, all interview processes involve some amount of personal investment, and if applying for multiple jobs it will be harder to prepare in the necessary detail. And if, unfortunately, you are repeatedly unsuccessful this rejection may test your motivation and resilience.

Alternatively, you may select specific roles for which to apply. Employers already receive large numbers of applications for most jobs, and so to save them and you time it may be preferable to only apply for specific jobs. Your performance in the interview might also be better because you feel greater commitment and affinity to the post for which you are applying and will have had more opportunity to find out about the role and be better able to speak meaningfully about it and answer questions more effectively.

When choosing a job, some practical considerations need to be made. First of all, read the description of the post and consider is this a job that you would enjoy doing? Is the work repetitive and routine, or challenging and complex? Some people enjoy working in an established pattern and within strict protocols or guidelines, with close supervision and high levels of interaction with other members of the multi-disciplinary team (MDT). Others prefer a high degree of change and unpredictability. Some working environments have a large amount of lone or autonomous working, while others involve team-working. It is important to think about the nature of the work and what you are required to do, and whether this suits your personal disposition, preference and skill set. It is worth bearing in mind that when in training you have spent a long time regularly moving to different clinical environments and you may have become accustomed to regular change. Unless you are applying for a rotational post, the role for which you are applying will not change unless you acquire another job and so it is necessary to consider whether your interest in the post will endure.

Think back to your previous practice placements.

- Consider the setting you felt most comfortable in during your placements.
- Now identify the factors that led you to feel this way. For example, you might have liked the autonomy and working with patients in their own homes that comes with working in the community. Or alternatively, you may have preferred being part of a large team, and working in the more scientific and technological environment in the hospital wards.
- Think about how your preference matches with you as a person in terms of your attributes and personality. For example, people that are quietly confident and evaluators by nature may thrive in the community, while those who are team players enjoy ward-based settings and the close proximity of colleagues.
- Neither preference – for the community or an inpatient setting – is necessarily the right answer, as we are all different. Instead it is important that we work in an environment that complements our disposition and personality.

Activity 2.1

THE JOB SPECIFICATION: ESSENTIAL AND DESIRABLE CHARACTERISTICS

If at this point you are still interested in the post, go on and read the person specification. Look at the essential characteristics, and those that are desirable and consider how you might meet these. In nearly all jobs in the description there will be a list of essential and desirable characteristics. As the words suggest, essential characteristics are mandatory, while desirable characteristics are more flexible and optional criteria.

Often the wording of job specifications can feel quite sophisticated and high-powered. You may read the essential attributes of the job specification and go from feeling as though you really want the job to doubting whether you can ever meet the requirements. It may help to discuss the post with a good friend, mentor, peer, tutor, or someone you trust and who knows you well to consider how you might meet the requirements, and which aspects of your experience match these attributes. When going through the essential and desirable characteristics write down how you meet these, as this will be useful for your application. If in the interview you can clearly and concisely explain exactly how you meet the essential specifications, this will satisfy the interviewer's curiosity and make the interview a more pleasant experience, and is likely to help your chances of success. In order to prove that you are suited to the role, you will need to meet all of the essential characteristics. This is why it helps to discuss your application with someone else, as often these criteria include so many aspects of the person it may exhaust your capacity to answer all of them in new ways. Someone else may provide a fresh perspective to add to your own self-perception.

Although the role of a qualified nurse may appear to be demanding, reassuringly nursing roles are set within a structure, and a Band 5 staff nurse post has clear and specific expectations (see below) within the structure of line management and seniority. Those roles at the higher grades involve a high level of authority, expertise, management responsibility and scope.

If you are able to clearly meet as many of the desirable characteristics as possible as well as all of the essential characteristics it is likely you will be a good candidate for the role for which you are applying. The non-mandatory and more flexible nature of the desirable characteristics also means that they may be met more adaptably. However, ensure that any achievement, attribute or skill that you use in meeting the desirable characteristics is consistent with what is required and not an exaggeration. How you describe yourself in relation to the desirable characteristics allows the interviewer or person reading your application to appreciate you as an individual and is sometimes used by employers to decide between applicants where they are closely matched in terms of overall competence.

RESEARCH INTO THE JOB

It is also important to find out what the job involves, and what it is really like. The best-case scenario is that you will have some direct knowledge and understanding of the clinical area. This may be through having been on placement there, even more than once. Also consider whether this was early in your training or later on. This is because your understanding of the clinical area may be more realistic if you have been there later in your training where you took more responsibility and were more involved in the delivery of care. This may not exclusively be the case.

If you have always been a very diligent, observant and perceptive student you may have been placed in the area early in your training and have gained a good perspective of what it might be like to work there. Alternatively, you may have worked on the clinical area through the bank, or on the agency. It is possible that the clinical area may be well known and have a good reputation. Alternatively, you may have seen the post in an advert, online, or in a nursing journal or you may know staff that work on the area or have friends or family with knowledge and experience of that clinical area. It may be that the unit or areas you apply to follows a clinical specialism that is the same as somewhere you carried out a placement while on training and is in another part of the country. This means you may have fewer sources of information on which to proceed than in other cases, so you might want to phone a named contact on the advert or visit to get a feel for the place and meet prospective colleagues. Being proactive and finding out about a job creates a positive impression upon an employer but do not rely upon this. You may have visited and the staff may have liked you, but if you deliver a poor interview, having visited is unlikely to get you the job on its own.

Think about the area where you are applying to work.

- Consider how you heard about the vacancy. If this is from placement experience, whether this was earlier or later in the course. If this was early in the course, you might have less insight into the work of the unit than if you had a placement later in the course when your knowledge level was greater.
- Think about what you know about the specific clinical area and whether you have heard other people's opinions about what it is like.
- If the work of the area is a specialism, you may have written a theory assignment on this during the course, or have undertaken some reading about this area of expertise, or it may have been the subject of your dissertation.

Activity 2.2

Box 2.1   Role and responsibility of a Band 5 nurse

- Provide care of a high standard consistent with local and national policy.
- Deliver care for specific groups of patients.
- Be responsible for a caseload of patients, yet with indirect supervision from a senior nurse.

(Continued)

(Continued)

- Assess, plan, implement and evaluate care, implement care plans and apply the nursing process.
- Support the learning of junior staff, including students and unregistered practitioners.
- Act as a practice supervisor for student nurses.
- Collaborate with the MDT to advance patient care.
- Engage in the promotion of the health and wellbeing of patients.
- Foster family-centred care and actively support carers, family and significant others.
- Organise, plan and monitor patient care.
- Work within teams and actively coordinate and delegate care.
- Promote patient safety.
- Enhance the quality of patient care.

Source: adapted from Forde-Johnston, 2018

The more sources of information you have the better. But consider what supports your opinion and ensure that you want to work there for the right reasons, and that your expectations are realistic. Some clinical areas with very good reputations and high standing may be difficult to work at, whether this is due to the negative aspects not being noticed or tolerated because the clinical area has other strong positive aspects. Or the leadership may have undergone a change for the worse, or it may just not be the right environment for you to choose as your first job. Alternatively, a workplace can simply 'feel right'. The culture of a workplace is tangible and palpable. We frequently feel it as soon as we walk onto a ward or into an office. However, at the same time it is very hard to quantify. What is perceived as a good workplace and a positive, supportive environment varies, as we are all different, with subjective preferences and needs. We spend a lot of time at work and feeling that you *'fit in'* is important if you are to enjoy your job.

Activity 2.3

Early on in qualified practice we often need quite close support and reassurance so that we know we are doing the job correctly. But some people need more, or a different form of support than others.

Think about your support needs.

- These might include clinical supervision, for example for an hour every week.
- Or shadowing other qualified nurses, in order to see and learn from different leadership styles.
- Or specific learning related to the specialist practice of the clinical area where you are applying.

In **Chapter 4** of the book, we discuss the importance of good preceptorship in your first job. Yet it is especially important that you have a good experience in the early stages of post-qualified practice. If you are to deliver the best care that you can and find your work rewarding and fulfilling, it is necessary that you agree with the prevailing philosophy and culture of the workplace and feel accepted and valued by other team members. Working alongside other capable and dynamic nurses whose beliefs and values you also share will allow you to learn in an environment which feels safe and supportive and will promote your own growth and professional development.

Likewise working in an area where there are problems with recruitment and low morale may expose you to workplace stress and difficult situations for which you may feel ill-equipped. Even though you may be qualified as a new registrant, it is essential to have support during the early stages of post-qualified practice in order to effectively withstand the demands that this places upon you. Ironically, in areas where there are challenges in delivering effective care, such as staff shortages, there is also commonly the absence of a culture of support, which the Francis Report (2013) tells us further compounds unacceptable standards of care.

Often, students do not believe that clinical areas in their locality which are known for poor standards might be the subject of for example a CQC (Care Quality Commission) report, or even television documentary. However, it is worth remembering that nursing is nationwide, and all areas are subject to inspection. This does also mean that while there may be clinical environments with unacceptable standards, there may also be areas of excellence. It is important to find a first job in an area where the standards are high and the values and principles of your peers, colleagues and managers reflect your own. As with the choices we make about our close personal relationships and friendships, it is necessary to take responsibility and make informed choices about where we apply to work.

CURRICULUM VITAE (CV)

A curriculum vitae or CV is a record of your career to date, and a summary of your professional background, learning and relevant information about you and your career to date. A CV reflects your achievements, skills, training and learning and will give a prospective employer a good idea of who you are. Often people are confused about how much or how little to write, and what to include. A prospective employer may receive anything from tens to hundreds of applications or more, and needs to be able to read them quickly. If the CV is too long, too personalised, information is hard to find, or if it is poorly laid out and formatted it is likely to be discarded, no matter how suitable the applicant. Therefore, it is time well spent devoting some time to developing a good CV. Often it is suggested that a CV is no more than one A4 page in length. It is challenging, and difficult to encapsulate a lifetime of experience onto one page; however, there are many templates available to use, or you may create your own.

Bear in mind that you want to create an instant and professional impression, and so avoid excessive adornment, or a style which is very personal, idiosyncratic or elaborate. While the CV is all about you, at the same time it ought to convey a profile of you as a professional. Your CV ought to reflect some element of personality, but a central intention has to be to convey the impression of you as a reliable and responsible professional. Therefore, use a formal type font such as Times New Roman or Ariel with headings in bold type font. Begin with your name, contact details and date of birth, and then follow with a simple but clear structure, such as: professional training, employment history, education and learning, skills and interests. Each of these areas is discussed next.

Professional training

This needs to come first, as the CV is being produced to support your application for a professional nursing role. It is necessary to include the date(s) of your training, and any other nursing related or professional courses you have studied.

Employment history

Include all periods of employment, beginning with the most recent, and going back in time. If you have had more than one part-time job simultaneously include them in chronological order with the one where you worked the longest listed first. Include voluntary work and internships in the skills and interests section. Often applicants do not mention these experiences, yet they sometimes add an important extra attribute to your application and demonstrate important learning and experience. Where there are gaps in your employment history, provide an explanation. If you became a full-time student, mention this and refer to the next section.

Education and learning

Include formal education only from A level, as you only have a limited amount of space. If for example you received good grades in a language or have a flair for learning other languages, you might want to expand on this skill in what you say in the section which follows.

Skills and interests

In this section it is important to include capabilities such as your most recent Disclosure and Barring Service (DBS) check, whether you have a driver's licence, whether you are computer literate and other specialist skills. Any that are especially related to the role will help. But importantly these demonstrate that you are a responsible person. Whether you can speak another language and any other skills and abilities that you may have are also worth mentioning together with voluntary work, internships and whether you have travelled, for example.

Interests are healthy and necessary, and it is important to demonstrate that you are a rounded person and have a work–life balance. Many people feel that their leisure activities are not especially different or interesting compared to those of other people. Yet interests such as home baking, family history or sewing are just as good (and safer) than rock climbing, snowboarding or extreme sports. However, if you still doubt the value of this section imagine your application, and then your application without mentioning any interests. Employers want staff who can switch off and recharge their batteries; having leisure interests shows that you have a personality and character and adds breadth to your application. Often the value of the skills and interests' section of an application is underestimated. While on its own it will not secure you the job, if I am a busy interviewer and have seen a number of similarly skilled people for a job, I may remember a person due to their interest or hobby and form a positive impression of them.

The personal statement

The process of making a job application varies, but often there is an online application form which includes your details and demographic data. NHS Jobs (www.jobs.nhs.uk/cgi-bin/advsearch) is a free online resource that is user friendly and time efficient and allows you to populate a form that you can then use for applications to different jobs. However, remember to regularly update your information in case your details change. For most jobs, to make an application you will be required to complete an online application form, submit a CV, and write a personal statement or cover letter and nominate referees. So, when applying for a job, think of people who may be suitable choices for referees. Generally, it is required that a referee needs to have known you for a minimum of two years. Out of courtesy always ask your referee in advance. This will ensure that they will be aware that a reference request can be expected and begin to think about what to say about you if they do not know already. Also, if they are going on holiday in the near future, or are likely to be absent for some time they can let you know so that you can ask someone else if a more urgent response is required. For your first job after qualifying it makes sense to ask your personal tutor from university. For a second referee though, and for jobs you apply for in the future, choose a nurse qualified in the same branch of nursing as you, and with whom you have worked with as your senior or manager; they can provide a credible account of your skills and competencies as a practitioner.

The personal statement should not just be seen as a means of gaining you access to the interview. Instead it is part of an interlinked process together with your interview and any other stages that there may be to the selection process. The personal statement needs to be authentic and to represent you as a person and professional. At the interview the discussion adds to this impression and reassures the interviewers that you are the person you describe yourself to be. This is difficult, as on the one hand you do not want to undersell yourself and be honest in answering questions to the point of compromising or contradicting yourself, but at the same time it is important to be very genuine and honest. Therefore, practising answering interview questions is invaluable in helping you explain your understanding of professional practice in relation to the questions you are asked.

Write a different statement for each job that you apply for. While your skills and attributes are the same, you will be applying different aspects of these in each role. Furthermore, every job will be different, and employers will be flattered to know that you have taken the time to find out about the specific features of their ward, clinical area, Trust or organisation. Begin your statement with a broad and general comment, and then narrow down to the specifics. Base your points on the specifications stated in the advert, starting with those that are essential and followed by those that are desirable. Address them in the same order as they appear in the person specification. If you find you meet all of the essential attributes and most of those that are desirable already you may well be applying for a job for which you are very well suited. However, no one ever meets all of the requirements. At some points you may feel you are stretching to meet these criteria. In your mind consider how you might answer an interviewer's question with regards to how closely you really do meet this aspect. What have you done in your life and what skills or competencies do you possess that might meet this attribute, or at least mean that you might quickly be able to learn or acquire this knowledge? Astute interviewers will focus on areas where an applicant does not seem to meet the personal criteria of the job. This does not mean that if you do not completely meet all of the essential attributes you will not get the job. Part of the process is to identify how individuals that are different might fit into a role. However, if you cannot find anything about yourself that meets an essential requirement and friends and colleagues cannot suggest anything then you might want to consider whether to apply.

Once you have written your application, print off a copy and read it through as though you were looking at someone else's work. Consider the limitations or comments which you might question or want to ask more about. Think of how you might answer these questions. You might also make notes on what you would say. Once you have completed your application keep a copy that is easily retrievable and read it again before the interview, as there may be some time between your completing the application and the interview and you may forget what you have written. This is because much of the information that your interviewers have about you will come from what you have written on this application and it will inform the questions that they ask you, if the selection process allows.

THE INTERVIEW

Interviews can be anxiety-provoking and stressful experiences. Yet we need them as a transparent and open competitive process, so that roles are fairly attributed based on suitability and competence. It may be a stressful experience but the boost that can be gained from being successful in an interview will enhance your sense of esteem and self-confidence and you will have the satisfaction of knowing that you have earned the role. Most job application processes will involve an interview, whether this is with two people, or a panel of several or more. To reduce the potential for bias, interviews often use the same questions, and in some cases specific interviewers ask the same question(s) of each applicant. Furthermore, the performance of applicants is generally assessed in relation to the job specification and the essential and desirable characteristics of the post-holder as objective criteria against which your performance can be measured, and decisions justified. Yet any encounter between people, even where there are multiple interviewers, has the possibility of involving subjective influences or bias. Often the possibility of subjectivity is mitigated by the use of other additional methods that will provide an indication of the applicant's suitability in certain aspects of the role, such as:

- Competency tasks
- Scenario-based tests
- Written tests, including drug calculation tests
- Presentations on a set theme
- The use of test centres and online tests.

Looking at the above, identify which you are good at.

If you really wanted a job, but the selection process involved a method you were not good at, or you felt you could not do, do you think you might decide to not apply?

If you answered *'yes'* you may lose out on a job you would really like, just because of the method of selection.

If you said *'no'*, what if you tried to overcome your fears and limitations and practised at the selection method but were still unsuccessful?

Activity 2.4

We only develop and expand our skill set by undertaking new tasks which we have not previously carried out. Sometimes this is challenging and exposes our limitations, but working with our motivation and personal perspective enables us to become more adaptable and resilient when carrying out tasks that we find difficult. Being positively motivated and working to reduce our doubts and fear means that we avoid creating self-fulfilling prophecies, and rather than thinking ourselves into failing, we can instead use motivation to create success, or at the very least improve our chances. Of course, there are some situations and tasks which exceed our capabilities. Especially in clinical practice it is necessary to work within our own scope of practice (NMC 2018). In this case, in an interview situation or as part of a selection process, it is helpful to know how, and in what ways, we fall short, and consider how we might develop to ensure future success. As a qualified nurse having undergone and succeeded at professional training it is reasonable to expect that you will succeed at the interview and selection process, unless there are problems with your preparation. Therefore, if you experience repeated failure it is even more important to seek feedback, and to look for patterns, where the same issues emerge as problems. We ought not to fear failure but instead we should be wary of how our fears can prevent us from trying to access new opportunities and learning (Jeffers, 2011).

Interviews have numerous benefits. They represent a good chance to learn more about yourself, develop the ability to respond to questions that you might not expect, function in situations where you do not feel in control, and to improvise and cope under pressure. These skills will be useful, for example when working with patients whose health status changes suddenly, or when responding to and reassuring concerned carers, family or significant others who may be very worried about the patient. Having skills and experience in interviews will be useful in the future as it is likely that you will be required to attend further interviews if seeking other jobs or promotion, or applying for courses. Seeing the interview as a learning experience will help, as often how we feel can become determined by short-term goals and the most sig-nificant issue in our life at the time. Instead, if you can view your search and application for your first job in the wider context of your professional training and overall development you may be less moved by short-term worries and anxieties.

When preparing for an interview, consider the following points:

- **Read the instructions** you have been given very carefully, as you may be required to prepare something in advance.
- **Do some reading** in advance of the interview about policy and guidance relating to the clinical area where you are applying but also more broadly. Think about issues pertaining to professional conduct, and any current themes that are being discussed in the media
- **Consider commonly encountered** clinical scenarios, ethical dilemmas or problems relating to the clinical area where you are applying. This will help you to prepare for any scenario-related questions
- **Think about the scope of the role** for which you are applying and how you might demonstrate your willingness and ability to take responsibility. But also consider working within the scope of your competence and the need to demonstrate your ability to work as a team member
- **Be aware of commonly encountered interview questions** (see below) and know the answers that you would give to these.

Preparing for the interview is not just about wearing appropriately smart clothes; you also need to plan your journey to the venue well in advance and in detail. If it is somewhere you have never been to before, make sure you know the route, and if possible, make a visit before the date of the interview, so you know the locality and where to go. If appropriate, know where you will park. If the interview is being held some distance away from where you live and in a busy location that you may struggle to get to first thing in the morning it might be easier to travel down and stay overnight beforehand. This will allow you to focus on your preparation for the interview, as opposed to being preoccupied with other distractions such as finding your location when in busy traffic.

There are only a finite number of questions which can be asked in an interview. Scenario-related questions are difficult, and it tends to be the case that you can either answer them or not, as these rely upon specific knowledge and an awareness of procedure. However, if you have prepared well then you should not be caught out by a scenario-based question if it is reasonable and realistic. In some cases, scenarios will conform to regularly encountered dilemmas specific to the clinical area. It should be expected that you ought to be able to answer a scenario-based question, as these scenarios will happen in the job for which you are applying. However, in some cases where you have not encountered the scenario before, it is possible to solve it by thinking logically about the situation, considering the circumstances and advantages and disadvantages of each course of action before making a final decision.

Together with a friend, agree on a specific job and clinical area, and practise asking each other the following questions:

- Why do you want this job?
- What skills and competencies do you feel you bring to this role?
- Why should we employ you?

Activity 2.5

Think about the answers, and perhaps write them down and build a repertoire of responses. However, be careful not to just learn these by rote, as sometimes questions are a composite, or a slight variation of other questions, and so you may need to adapt the content of your response to effectively answer the question; it is necessary to be able to demonstrate your ability to think quickly and improvise.

Perhaps the most difficult questions are what are your strengths and weaknesses. Table 2.1 gives some examples of strengths and weaknesses. You might find it useful to think about what are your own strengths and weaknesses. Even though weaknesses are perceived as being problematic, everyone has them, and so it is a question that we can all answer. In fact, not being able to identify a weakness is more of a concern, as this might be seen as demonstrating an absence of self-knowledge and awareness.

The answers to the questions in Table 2.1 are all realistic and might apply to many newly qualified nurses applying for their first job. They will allow a prospective employer to understand your limitations but also appreciate your capabilities. Being sure of your weaknesses can be seen as a strength. It represents

Table 2.1   Personal strengths and weaknesses

Question	Possible answer
What are your strengths?	• I can often analyse situations very quickly and see answers to problems
	• I am a good team player and enjoy working with others and strive to get the most out of my colleagues
	• I am enthusiastic, keen and eager to learn
What are your weaknesses?	• I struggle to delegate as I lack confidence
	• I will need support in preceptorship in administering medication
	• While I have gained clinical experience on practice placements I had not worked in nursing until commencing the course. Therefore I need more practice experience

self-awareness, honesty and maturity. Perhaps most importantly, identifying your weaknesses clearly and specifically will allow an employer to know how to help you in practice. Employers know that no one is perfect and appreciate interviewees who are specific and clear on their shortcomings. This saves the interviewer needing to figure out vague or unclear answers. Or even worse, responses that are not genuine.

In the interview remember to be yourself. Often interviewees give answers to questions with an astute awareness of wanting to create a positive impression. That is understandable, as you want to get the job. However, sometimes interviewees give answers they do not believe. Once you begin to do this it becomes difficult as not only are you thinking of the answer to give to questions but filtering it as well to check that it is consistent with the persona you are creating. Most interviewers are well used to reading people and can see this going on and feel unconvinced. Therefore, the best approach is to be yourself. At the same time, it is important to try, as in some cases interviewees can go to the reverse extreme and take the maxim of *'what you see is what you get'* too far. While honesty is good, be aware you are in an interview and a certain professional air is expected.

Having suggested that you be yourself it is worth remembering that even in community settings nurses always work in teams. We discuss this further in **Chapter 7**. However, in an interview remember to consider the importance of promoting team-working. I suggest this as sometimes in interviews newly qualified nurses emphasise their use of their own skills and capabilities at the expense of involving the wider team. This can create an impression of the newly qualified nurse as not being aware of the importance of team-working or of being preoccupied with their own performance. While interviewers are keen to see the capabilities of the interviewee and it is important to show your capabilities as an autonomous practitioner, be aware of demonstrating a broad range of capabilities.

The interview ought to be a hospitable and maybe even pleasant experience. Most interviewers are friendly and responsive and will place you at your ease and make you welcome. If not, you might want to consider whether you want the job. To be effective interviews ought to be two-way, with the interviewer responding to the interviewee, as opposed to being blank and inert. In the actual interview if you do not know the answer to a question admit it as opposed to trying to front it out and use bravado. Answers such as *'I don't know that but will look it up later'* demonstrate transparency and openness. Not knowing the answer to a question might not be fatal to your chances. Yet depending on whether you might reasonably have been expected to know the answer to the question you might want to reflect on the effectiveness of your preparation and what you might do differently in preparing for future interviews.

If you leave the interview convinced you have got the job it is possible that you are correct. However, I have often known interviewees give an excellent interview, and come away feeling that they were unsuccessful. Some people dwell on mistakes, even if small, or the things they did not say, yet do not credit the many positive things that they may have said. After an interview it is often hard to know whether we have got the job or not. Therefore, resist the temptation to rake over the coals and go over your performance. But it is hard to resist, and if however, you do, perhaps for every negative aspect that you think of also consider a positive aspect of your performance. If you are in competition with friends for the same vacancies bear in mind that other people's accounts of their performances are often inaccurate or exaggerated, and sometimes people say things to make themselves feel better or bolster fragile confidence. People who do less well often overestimate their impact, while those who are modest and may say they did badly might have impressed. Then there are those in the middle. Either way, listening to our competitors can often lead us to make detrimental comparisons which can be incorrect.

AFTER THE INTERVIEW: FEEDBACK

Applying for a job always involves risk, as for most job vacancies there are more qualified applicants and good interviewees than are appointed. The best-case scenario though is that you are successful and get the job. Often if you are told in a phone call, and normally from someone from the interview panel, it is likely that they will tell you what aspects of your performance gained you the job. It is worth thinking about the feedback and considering whether this corresponds with your own impressions about what was good about your interview. Even though your interview was successful there are always things to be learned, and bearing in mind that it is highly likely that you will be in interviews in the future, it is worth considering what else you can develop.

If you have not gained the post, even though it might seem to be futile if it is not volunteered it is worth asking for feedback. However, to begin with it is necessary to attend to personal feelings. Jobs enhance our lives. If you are unsuccessful it is hard not to feel upset for several reasons. Applying and preparing for an interview is time consuming and involves effort and commitment, which may then seem to have been for no purpose. You may have already been contemplating the opportunity this could have provided to gain new skills and develop personally and professionally. While it can feel like a personal slight and that this reflects upon you as a person, it is worth realising logically, even if you still feel emotionally hurt, that the judgement is made on your suitability for the role as a professional and is not about you as a person. Allow yourself to experience these feelings, and recognise them, as it is important that we *'own'* and accept these.

Even though you may be tempted to move forward and forget the experience, feedback is always available. The interviewers will have assessed your interview and application against criteria and have documented their decision and the reasons and you have a right to ask for feedback on your interview. Therefore, even if it is not offered, it is reasonable to request feedback on your performance at the interview. Frequently there is a high volume of applications for jobs, and the number of applicants invited to interview can vary, with sometimes high numbers of people invited. Therefore, not being automatically offered feedback may simply be due to resources. Feedback can take various forms, ranging from letters to phone calls, although speaking directly to someone, and ideally a member of the interview panel, will provide the most detailed perspective. When receiving feedback interpret what is said in relation to your perception of your performance and synthesise these accounts. It may be something that you recognise from previous feedback from placements or other job interviews. If so, reflect upon why this is a repeated issue. However, as well as receiving and understanding feedback, if we are to change things in the future it is necessary to identify learning and action points and consider what you might do to change and enhance your future performance.

It may unfortunately be the case that you gave a good interview, but another candidate was outstanding on the day. From long experience of being involved with many interview panels for different types of role and post, it is common for one applicant to shine on the day and eclipse the other candidates. This can be hard to take for other applicants who may also have been perfectly suited for the job. In this situation it is important to think about how you feel, to try and take some comfort from knowing that you were good enough but just not quite equal to the successful applicant and then move on as quickly as possible. Often this situation can reaffirm your confidence, as you know that in all likelihood you will get the next, or another, vacancy very soon.

In the fullness of time, and in hindsight, not getting a job can sometimes be seen to be the right thing. Perhaps the vacancy was not one to which your skills and aptitudes were suited. Experiencing disappointment can become useful in supporting other colleagues experiencing the same feelings in future. Furthermore, if you are ever in the position of needing to turn an applicant down, you will be able to empathise with them. We all experience setbacks in life in many different ways but confronting these takes honesty and genuine courage and makes us better people.

Your first job as a qualified nurse is perhaps more important than you realise. As time passes it will gain in significance. While there are certain considerations that can be made, and when job hunting it helps to think carefully about the vacancies for which you apply, there are only so many factors you can manage or situations you can anticipate. In practice, learning occurs through doing and proceeding based upon what we know but then stopping to reflect upon the results of our actions in order to see the way forward.

Therefore, the skills of nursing can be applied to the process of job-seeking. It is important when looking back to not have regrets, and perhaps worth bearing in mind that we do not make mistakes. We may get things wrong and make poor or unwise choices but at the time those decisions all seemed reasonable based on what we knew, and, if in the same position again we would do exactly the same thing. Therefore, do not over-prepare, expect the perfect vacancy to appear, or be hard on yourself for a perceived failure or mistake. Success or failure in an interview or job selection process rarely depends upon a huge margin. Often selection processes are multi-staged and rely upon you creating an impression in several different formats or media, which is established, affirmed and then reaffirmed. Therefore, minor errors are of minimal consequence and exert little impact upon the final result. And so getting or not getting a job depends upon larger issues such as our overall approach, communication or interpersonal skills generally, and our values and beliefs, as opposed to an incautious remark. In this respect the process of finding a job is a useful reflective activity in confirming who you are but also your values, strengths, skills and limitations as a qualified practitioner.

REFERENCES

Forde-Johnston, C. (2018). *How to Thrive as a Newly Qualified Nurse*. Banbury: Lantern Publishing.

Francis, R. (2013). Report of the Mid Staffordshire NHS Foundation Trust Public Inquiry. London: The Stationery Office.

Jeffers, S. (2011). *Feel the Fear and Do It Anyway*. London: Arrow Books.

NHS Jobs (2019). www.jobs.nhs.uk/cgi-bin/advsearch, accessed 7 April 2019.

Nursing and Midwifery Council (NMC) (2018). *The Code: Professional Standards of Practice and Behaviour for Nurses, Midwives and Nursing Associates*. www.nmc.org.uk/standards/code/, accessed April 2019.

3

Becoming a qualified nurse

Nick Wrycraft

'How nurses think and feel about themselves as nurses evolves throughout their lifetime; however, the years of education and training are vital in shaping the trajectory and nature of their professional identities. It is during this time that an individual develops from a lay person into a nurse, acquiring the knowledge, skills and attributes of a professional.'

(Johnson et al. 2012: 566)

Training to become a nurse represents a sustained and enduring demonstration of commitment and perseverance. Anyone who reaches that point deserves respect purely for having arrived there. Yet when achieving that goal, it can be hard to temper the pride and sense of achievement with the knowledge that as one journey ends another begins.

Learning outcomes

- The transition from being a student to a newly qualified nurse.
- How the completing student can prepare themselves for the challenges ahead.
- A concept of time that incorporates experience in contributing to transition.

It can be difficult to know how to feel when qualifying as a nurse. This milestone for many people ranks alongside other significant life events and is something with regard to which we may experience deeply felt emotions. One student described it to me as follows: 'Qualifying as a nurse is the best thing that ever happened to me.' While this may be thought of as a spontaneous comment made in the moment, these words were spoken seven months after the person qualified, and having just secured a promotion, been accepted onto an educational course, and with the guarantee of their new salary being able to secure a mortgage on a newly built house. In light of these events their comment may seem entirely proportionate. Nursing has given this person's life direction, purpose and a sense of fulfilment which they told me at earlier points in time even they might never have expected.

This recently qualified nurse's rapid progress and success is exceptional, and I have included it only to illustrate just what qualifying as a nurse can do for your career and life. Success is not only measured in progression, promotion and upwards career trajectory. If you are still working as a staff nurse face-to-face with patients twenty years after qualifying, you will have succeeded. Perhaps most important of all is to derive fulfilment from your work. Nursing involves working with people. This is evident in team-working, supporting students and learners, and most important of all delivering effective care to patients. Often nursing is a career considered to be a vocation, and the notion of serving others and improving the quality of the lives of patients is a powerful motivating factor and benefit in itself. Yet the notion of vocation and the interconnection between professional values and personal commitment is a powerful intertwining of personal commitment and the acquisition of a professional perspective. The process of training and developing and acquiring this identity is worth reflecting upon, so that we know not only where we have arrived at but how we got there.

This chapter should be read as an exploration in clarifying your thoughts pertaining to where you are now but also in deciding where to go next. We will discuss the structure for student support and learning in the practice area. Within this framework the newly qualified nurse can both contribute to supporting and promoting student learning, while simultaneously developing their own knowledge and skills. The discussion then progresses to consider the relationship between self-concept and professional identity, and how these notions explain the process of your professional socialisation through your training. The chapter concludes by looking at the steps you will take next as your career develops.

SUPPORTING STUDENTS IN PRACTICE

Changes in the NMC Code in 2018 (NMC 2018a) amended the system for supporting students in practice commencing from September 2019. These have not essentially changed from the contents of the previous Code (NMC 2015) but were prompted by a need to adapt to the changing nature of the nursing workforce. For example, nursing assistants are to be included on the professional register (NMC 2018a). Yet for the purposes of this discussion the most significant change was to enhance the support students receive while learning in practice through the creation of the roles of practice supervisor, practice assessor, academic assessor and practice learning coordinators; though this last role is not specifically named in the revised Code (NMC 2018a) (see Figure 3.1).

These roles are identified by the NMC (2018b) as follows:

The Practice Supervisor (PS) is a registered professional who acts as a role model and monitors students' progress and development in the practice setting. In relation to assessment, the practice supervisor documents the student's performance with regard to the performance of practice competencies and conduct (Hoy and George 2018). Practice supervisors are likely to be staff that have not been qualified for a long period of time and are gaining experience, having prepared for this role by for example a brief workshop, or online training.

The Practice Assessor (PA) for nurses is a currently registered professional with the NMC. Although they are not necessarily from the same branch as the student, they must have relevant and suitable experience. It is necessary for them to be properly prepared and supported, and they observe and assess the student in practice in relation to their competencies. The practice assessor cannot simultaneously be the same student's practice supervisor but may supervise another student. The practice assessor carries out the student's summative assessment in liaison with the academic assessor and liaising with and using the practice supervisor's recorded feedback on the student's performance.

The Academic Assessor (AA) is a registered practitioner with the NMC, again not necessarily from the same nursing branch as the student, and is suitably prepared and supported. The academic assessor confirms the student's achievement with the practice assessor. It is also required that the academic assessor changes during the student's training, so that no one academic is the student's supervisor for the duration of their training.

Practice Learning Coordinator (PLC). The NMC also requires that a nominated person acts as a point of contact for students, offers support for students and can respond to their concerns and liaises with practice supervisors and assessors where necessary.

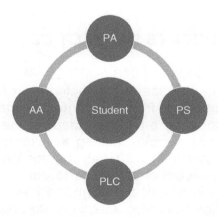

Figure 3.1   Supporting roles for nursing students in practice from September 2019

This model of support offers a comprehensive network of learning relationships for students. There is likely to be the opportunity for the student to learn facilitated by the practice supervisor in a flexible, supportive relationship which has the potential to foster genuine development, progress and team-working. However, there is a danger that the practice assessor is in a position of making decisions about the student's capabilities, while arguably not being the person best situated to make such judgements, as they do not know the student as well as the practice supervisor. Even though it is required that the practice supervisor record their observations of the student, and that they communicate with the practice assessor (Hoy and George, 2018) the form that this assumes is not described in the NMC guidance (2018b).

In addition, the nature of the role of the academic assessor in interacting with the practice assessor is also ambiguous, and arguably a misnomer with assessment possibly referring to the administration, as the practice assessor makes the final decision about the student's clinical competence. Essentially the success of this model relies upon effective and transparent communication, good relationships between the role holders, and a clear knowledge of the responsibilities and expectations of these positions. Potentially there is the opportunity to develop a culture within nursing where team-working is consciously cultivated and developed as part of the socialisation of student nurses, while newly qualified nurses are supported to make the transition into experienced nurses who can pass on their knowledge and develop flexible teaching methods to also prepare the next generation of nurses.

A very positive opportunity offered by this model is that newly qualified nurses are permitted to actively contribute to students' learning experiences immediately on qualification and can gain valuable teaching experience from the commencement of their professional career. While it might be argued that in itself the practice supervisor role does not directly prepare newly qualified nurses to become practice assessors, within the guidance it is specified that preparation is required for practice assessors that reflects the substantial nature of the role. The first generation of practice assessors are likely to be drawn from highly experienced staff that are already very acquainted with educating students, but in the future within the new system a different culture of practice-based nurse education will emerge and develop a new culture and identity as this system becomes established.

SELF-CONCEPT AND PROFESSIONAL IDENTITY

Practice experience is essential in moulding nurses' identity. Johnson et al. (2012) discuss how students assimilate their pre-existent self-concept within their emerging professional identity. When undergoing undergraduate education as a student nurse we are required to consider how our inherent identity and values integrate and cohere with those of the profession we are joining. In this section of the chapter we will discuss both of these aspects, beginning with self-concept.

Our self-concept can be understood as how we see ourselves as an individual in our cognitive, physical and social attributes. Self-concept also concerns how we perceive ourselves in terms of awareness, confidence and esteem (Marsh and Scalas 2010). The significance of this is in terms of how we relate to and know ourselves. Essentially self-concept is our relationship with ourselves. A relationship with ourselves may seem like an unusual notion, but we all have an interior mental world, even if only in terms of the monologue of thoughts that we constantly experience. Often, we take this for granted, as representing self-evident truths about the world around us but it is intensely subjective and personalised.

If I tend to lack confidence or underestimate my skills this is likely to influence how I interact with others, what I choose to do and my estimation of my capabilities. My self-talk and subjective perception will be an unquestioned part of my mental landscape and what I assume to be true. The same is the case if in contrast I am over-confident and have an exaggerated appraisal of my own abilities. It is therefore necessary to align our subjective self-concept with the objective appraisal others might have about us. Hopefully during the course of your training, you have received feedback on your performance from many qualified nurses and other health care staff in a variety of clinical specialisms. Mixed together with the assessment of your professional performance on clinical placements are comments relating to you as a person and individual.

These will be different for everyone and refer to our personal values and priorities but also be evident in our professional practice. For example, it may have been said that you place the care of the patient above all other considerations and demonstrate compassion. Or that if you see something going wrong you will ensure that attention is brought to the matter and display courage. These comments, while seeming to be quite general, are individual and say something about us but also relate to the profession of nursing. Often our strengths are innate and feel natural. We do not have to work too hard at enacting them. However, in relation to attributes which are not innate we may need to work at these and expend some effort in cultivating and developing them.

In this respect self-awareness is a powerful tool, as if we know ourselves, we are able to mediate our views to adjust to situations that we encounter in practice. For example, if I lack confidence in my skills, if asked to do something I have not carried out often or am still learning I may experience anxiety. Alternatively, if I tend to be too confident, I may underestimate the task and preparation that I need to undertake and pay less attention to a situation than is necessary. There are clear implications for patient safety and the ability of the individual to work as an effective and functioning member of a team. Developing competence involves overcoming innate attributes of personality to become a functioning professional.

Experience in practice supports us in the form of tacit or experiential, multifaceted learning on an emotional and intellectual level but also in terms of learning the social norms of working in a profession. However, to be effective, learning in practice has to be focused and intentional and to be more than simply time spent time in practice and knowing that we have changed and developed but knowing exactly how and in what way we have learned. Throughout your pre-registration training you are likely to have been repeatedly encouraged to reflect and develop your self-awareness.

Think of an aspect of your personality that has been repeatedly remarked upon during your nursing placements.

- Think about when this was first mentioned, and recall how you felt. Sometimes the identification of our personal features can evoke deep-seated emotional responses.
- Consider whether you feel different about that now.
- Reflect on the change that you have undergone.
- Often over time we develop our ability to receive feedback. It may be that during the nursing course you have developed skills in receiving comments about your performance. If so, this represents professional development and personal growth.

Activity 3.1

Often it is assumed that the promotion of reflection and self-aware practice is an inevitable consequence and requirement of a higher education course being delivered at degree level. However, the standards of proficiency for qualified nurses (NMC 2018b) specifically exhort us to develop self-awareness and engage in reflection. Working with ourselves in this manner can be challenging, as often this process evokes feelings of vulnerability and deep-seated emotions, yet an important benefit to be derived is challenging our assumptions and preconceptions. This offers the potential of making us better at what we do and at the same time becoming better as people (Freshwater 2002; Healy and McSharry 2011).

In contrast, professional identity pertains to career, occupation or vocational choices, and relates to our perceived position in society. Factors such as our encounters with others and how we process experience are influential in how this is formed (Sutherland et al. 2010). Cho et al. (2010) and O'Brien et al. (2008) in their research studies have found an association between career choice, job satisfaction, positive nursing image and staff retention. The implication for nursing is very clear. Johnson et al. (2012) mention that perceptions of nursing, such as lacking prestige, and being underpaid and stressful work, may act as a disincentive for students to apply, and there may be low expectations of the role and limited motivation among those who do apply. If these notions are given credence and reaffirmed in students' experience while on placement this may detrimentally influence student motivation and retention, or even lead to nurses of the future being poor role models.

A student whom I was teaching described being on their first placement and asked by a qualified nurse why they were studying nursing when they could earn more working in a supermarket. The student discussed this experience in class and sought feedback from their group and me as the tutor. Among the issues which emerged during this discussion was that the reasons why a person comes into nursing are different than those which might lead a person to work in retail. Also, as a group we all agreed that respect and self-belief is generated from within. A conclusion from the discussion was that this reflects the low self-regard that the qualified nurse had of themselves. However, because the qualified nurse may perceive nursing to be a career of low value, this belief is not necessarily true, and the student ought not necessarily to agree with this opinion. However, negative attitudes have the power to be corrosive and toxic, especially when these are expressed to people who are learning and may not have had other experiences with which to compare these views. It has been identified that career choice and commitment are central attributes concerning the formation of professional identity (Kroger and Marcia, 2011). At this point there is a blurring of personal values and professional identity.

When applying to nurse education we have expectations and perceptions of the role. This is both in terms of the practical competencies and performance of the role but also what it is like to have that position. The expectations of the role of the nurse are quite clear and incontrovertible. *Future Nurse: Standards of Proficiency for Registered Nurses* (NMC 2018b) outlines seven platforms which represent the range of competence, knowledge and skills that a qualified nurse ought to possess (Table 3.1). This document is intended to both guide the educational curriculum for student nurses of all disciplines and also to inform the public about what they can reasonably expect.

Table 3.1   Standards of Proficiency for Registered Nurses

Platform	Characteristics of the nurse
1	Being accountable as a professional
2	Promoting health and preventing ill health
3	Assessing needs and planning care
4	Delivering and evaluating care
5	Leading and managing nursing care and working as part of a team
6	Contributing to safety and quality care
7	Coordinating patient care

Source: adapted from NMC, 2018b

Some of these competencies have clear, practical content, for example, assessing needs and planning care (number 3), and delivering and evaluating care (number 4). Other platforms are broader, and less easy to directly assess, for instance, acting accountably (number 1) as a professional, and leading and managing nursing care and working as part of a team (number 5). Numbers 1, 5 and 7 of the platforms rely significantly on communication and interaction with other people.

Wenger's 'communities of practice' model (1999) (see **Chapter 4**) has been highly influential in training practice-based professions and emphasises social-isation as a learning process within which students develop new skills socially as well as technically in the clinical setting supported by an academic and a clinician. This is resonant of the structure for learning described earlier, where there is a practice supervisor (PS), practice assessor (PA) and academic asses-sor (AA), all supporting the student in their learning. Benefits of this approach are the development of professional attitudes which harness personal values and virtues with professional attributes.

Placements in clinical practice will inevitably expose students to experiences they may find challenging or dispiriting. Having access to a supportive network as outlined in the student supervision arrangements will ensure that difficult experiences can be discussed, processed and understood in the context of the student's learning and development. As adults we learn differently than at earlier points in our lives, and inevitably when working with people as well as technical knowledge we undergo learning that relates to our feelings and emotions.

What was your understanding of the role of a nurse before you began your training?

During your clinical placements has your understanding of the role of the nurse changed? If so, how has it changed?

Can you recall in what situations this realisation occurred?

Is your understanding of the role of the nurse as something more or less valuable than before?

Activity 3.2

In learning to become a nurse it is possible that our motivation may be chal-lenged, and we may be required to question, alter or even reconstruct our values system based on these situations. When studying to become a nurse, we learn about how people experience health and ill health which can lead us to witness experiences and situations we may have never encountered or thought to be possible. This is all part of learning and something that we could not have antic-ipated. Many students begin their course with quite limited experience and learn in a rapidly moving environment at a fast rate over the course. In these circum-stances it is possible to be aware that we have changed, yet not exactly how and in what way. In the next section of this chapter we will discuss how you can optimise your learning and reflection on your previous experience but also begin to derive a sense of unity of your own development and progress.

TRANSITION AS A LEARNING EXPERIENCE

How have you learned over the duration of your nurse education so far? The notion that we incrementally develop at a gradual rate across the course of professional training seems to run counter to the experience of many people. Instead we often ruminate on challenges that impede our progress and percolate the information emerging with new understandings or advances in our knowledge. Reflecting back on my personal learning and growth of realisation I have made seemingly quite sudden progress in my knowledge at times. Though in hindsight there has been much rumination going on seemingly in the background pre-empting these advancements. In this section of the chapter we look at how we understand time. A consequence for us in learning is that we can best use experience by seeing how our past influences and guides our present and directs us into the future, and also see our experiences as representing a unified pattern of growth and progress.

For thousands of years physicists and philosophers have presented varying concepts of what time is. A landmark in our understanding of time is discussed by Rovelli (2018), who describes Isaac Newton's conception of time as linear and measurable, and divisible into sections that are equal and incremental. For Newton we can measure time as though it has an objective reality, and it can be seen as a road along which we have travelled so far, and which stretches inexorably into the distance as far as the horizon (Figure 3.2).

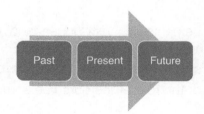

Figure 3.2   Newton's linear concept of time

Source: Wrycraft, 2017: 138

However, have you ever noticed that time seems to go faster when you are enjoying yourself but much slower when bored or not stimulated? This challenges the notion of time as being a uniform or consistent phenomenon. If a random group of people all agree to meet somewhere at a certain time, some will be present early, some will be exactly on time, and others late. Therefore, it appears that as individuals we have differing concepts of time and how it is to be managed. This also applies to us at different stages of our life. As a middle-aged man, days go much faster for me now than in my youth. While it might be claimed that this reflects our personal subjective perceptions, it also offers a useful insight into how time works. Time viewed almost as an objective entity that is amenable to specific and exact measurement seems to be illusory.

Rovelli (2018) refers to experiments conducted with very sensitive clocks that have identified differences in how time passes at varying altitudes leading to Newton's notion of temporality being open to doubt.

In contrast, Rovelli (2018) discusses Aristotle's view of time that was suggested more than a millennium before Newton's theory. For Aristotle, time depends on relations between objects and pertains to change, and in this sense, time can speed up or slow down, which explains how it appears to go more quickly when we are busy or having fun than when we are under-occupied or bored. We cannot dispute that time exists, because we age, and our lives have a beginning, duration and end, yet crucial for this debate is how we understand how time works. Rovelli (2018) points out that Newton's notion of time as being measurable in units and uniform has pervaded modern society, to the point of being unquestioningly accepted as true. However, I feel that this is unhelpful, and an incomplete appreciation of how we exist in time, which has the consequence of underestimating the value we can gain from our lived experience and limits our participation in truly reflective and self-aware practice.

Rovelli (2018) is careful to respect the views of both Newton and Aristotle, as they viewed time in quite different ways. For Newton time had a value as a unit of measurement; without watches and clocks and a calendar modern life would be challenging if not impossible, and so there is a use for Newton's perception. Yet Aristotle's view emphasises the value of time, and this leads me to a crucial point about how we exist in time. Martin Heidegger (2003) in a landmark work of philosophy published in 1927 entitled *Being and Time* wrote about the nature of time and how we exist within this phenomenon (depicted in Figure 3.3).

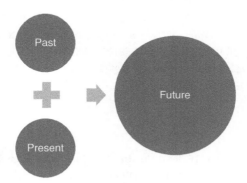

Figure 3.3   Heidegger's notion of time

Heidegger's (2003) notion of time challenges our prevailing Newtonian influenced perception of time as being linear. Within Heidegger's philosophy our past exists as a collection of memories and recollections derived from the experiences we have undergone, that is inaccessible to us, yet still with us in memories. This dense web of experience and reminiscences represents our sense of self and continuity, and the narrative of our life, yet is not a consistent and chronological record. For example, certain very brief periods of time may be of more worth and value to us than whole years or decades. The following lines from T.S. Eliot's poem *Burnt Norton* (1963) (from *Four Quartets*, first published in the United States in 1943) effectively capture this notion:

Time present and time past

Are both perhaps present in time future

And time future contained in time past.

Therefore, our experience of time represents a unity, where past and present and future converge, and our memories and experiences are held by us simultaneously with our present, and in the present we are the collection of our past. This lends a sense of coherence to our sense of identity. The consequence for our learning as nurses is that this places particular emphasis on the value of learned experience.

Activity 3.3

Think of a positive experience that you have had in your life and that you have remembered before or even frequently. Next, focus on a certain aspect of it that you have not previously thought about. So that for example if you normally focus on how a person looks, think about aspects of the environment of where you were. In recalling this experience you will remember more than you thought you did, as often remembering relies upon us recalling the same narrow and specific range of aspects of an experience. When we think about other parts of the event we realise that memory is actually more wide ranging than we ever thought. It may be that you are substituting certain details from imagination as opposed to memory but it is possible to recall things and even complete events which we felt that we had forgotten.

The implication of this for reflective learning is significant, and if we view time as overlapping the past and present, moving into the future as a concept, then there is the potential for us to learn more deeply from experience and develop further than if we perceive time as purely linear and chronological. Your repository of collected knowledge past and present intermingle to create a collective and continuous thread of existence. Heidegger (2003) emphasised living within the present. Yet reiterating his same arguments, I believe they instead point in a different direction, and that your student nurse education represents a vast resource for continued learning which will serve you well as you move forward into your qualified nursing future. Learning nursing involves confronting and coming to terms with aspects of human experience:

The starting point for learning is the encounter with the patient and his/her suffering. Receiving the patient's narrative is, according to the students', a reverent act. They show great respect for it as conversations with patients can create insecurity and fear. If the students do not get support in mastering this encounter with the patients, they will instead withdraw from the close proximity to the patient and observe the caring event from a distance.

(Ekebergh 2011: 386)

Yet at the same time as our life passes and we grow older our nursing knowledge becomes more resonant as we become aware of our own mortality. This is not necessarily a selfish thought, as it is inevitable that we will all age and experience frailty as we enter further stages of life; instead it is important to accept and embrace our experience, and as opposed to a selfish realisation this instead represents a realisation of our humanity.

A colleague once remarked to me that when they were training as a nurse there were some concepts which they could not see the value of at the time but that they later came to appreciate and understand. For me there has been much that I have learned in nursing that has gained greater depth of meaning and value as time has passed and I have gained in life experience. This is consistent with Erikson's ninth stage of the life cycle and much of the discussion in **Chapter 10**. In this respect the growth we undergo through our life experience becomes a self-defining pathway into our future. Regarding the past, present and future as inextricably connected can give a sense of unity to our learning, reinforce our sense of identity, and offer a fresh perspective for our future development.

In this chapter we have looked at your transition from being a senior student to a newly qualified nurse. Making this change may be eased by the new arrangements for student supervision. This will ensure that newly qualified nurses gain valuable experience through teaching and providing learning opportunities for students, yet without the responsibility for summatively assessing their overall competence. For newly qualified staff this offers a useful opportunity in making a measured transition to becoming experienced in nursing and capable of assessing student competence.

We have also looked at personal and professional identity and how these intertwine in contributing to the development of professional identity. What compels us to become nurses might also contribute to the professionals we become when translated to a practice context. Inevitably through clinical placements these values may become challenged and adapt or alter. Finally, we discussed how we can value what we learn through our concept of time.

REFERENCES

Cho, S.H., Jung, S.Y. and Jang, S. (2010). Who enters nursing schools and why do they choose nursing? A comparison with female non-nursing students using longitudinal data. *Nurse Education Today*, 30: 180–6.

Ekebergh, M. (2011). A learning model for nursing students during clinical studies. *Nurse Education in Practice*, 11: 384–9.

Eliot, T.S. (1963). *Collected Poems: 1909–1962*. London: Faber & Faber.

Freshwater, D. (ed.) (2002). *Therapeutic Nursing: Improving Patient Care through Self-Awareness and Reflection*. London: Sage Publications.

Healy, D. and McSharry, P. (2011). Promoting self-awareness in undergraduate nursing students in relation to their health status and personal behaviours. *Nurse Education in Practice*, 11: 228–33.

Heidegger, M. (2003). *Being and Time*. Oxford: Blackwell Publishing.

Hoy, G. and George, S. (2018). New standards on the supervision and assessment of students in practice. *Nursing Times*, 114(12): 27–9.

Johnson, M., Cowin, L.S., Wilson, I. and Young, H. (2012). Professional identity and nursing: contemporary theoretical developments and future research challenges. *International Nursing Review*, 59: 562–9.

Kroger, J. and Marcia, J.E. (2011). The identity statuses: origins, meanings and interpretations. In S.J. Schwartz, K. Luyckx and V.L. Vignoles (eds), *Handbook of Identity Theory and Research*, vol. 1. New York: Springer, pp. 31–53.

Marsh, H.W. and Scalas, L.F. (2010). Self-concept in learning: reciprocal effects model between academic self-concept and academic achievement. In P. Peterson, E. Baker and B. McGaw (eds), *International Encyclopedia of Education*. Oxford: Elsevier, pp. 660–7.

Nursing and Midwifery Council (NMC) (2015). *The Code: Professional Standard of Practice and Behaviour for Nurses and Midwives*. www.nmc.org.uk/standards/code/, accessed 22 September 2018.

Nursing and Midwifery Council (NMC) (2018a). *The Code: Professional Standards of Practice and Behaviour for Nurses, Midwives and Nursing Associates*. www.nmc.org.uk/standards/code/, accessed April 2019.

Nursing and Midwifery Council (NMC) (2018b). *Future Nurse: Standards of Proficiency for Registered Nurses*. www.nmc.org.uk/globalassets/sitedocuments/education-standards/future-nurse-proficiencies.pdf, accessed 16 March 2019.

O'Brien, F., Mooney, M. and Glacken, M. (2008). Impressions of nursing before exposure to the field. *Journal of Clinical Nursing*, 17: 1843–50.

Rovelli, C. (2018). *The Order of Time*. London: Allen Lane.

Sutherland, L., Howard, S. and Markauskaite, L. (2010). Professional identity creation: examining the development of preservice teachers' understanding of their work as teachers. *Teaching and Teacher Education*, 263: 455–65.

Wenger, E. (1999). *Communities of Practice: Learning, Meaning, and Identity*. Cambridge: Cambridge University Press.

Wrycraft, N. (2017). Taking practice forward through recovery. In N. Wrycraft and A. Coad (eds), *Recovery in Mental Health Nursing*. London: Open University Press/McGraw-Hill, pp. 128–43.

4

Preceptorship and supervision

Nick Wrycraft and Zoe Dodd

'The knowledge was there I just didn't feel that it was there and I didn't feel that I knew enough but then when I started talking about it and doing it and pulling things you know from wherever it was stored I thought "wow, I do know this", you know, "wow, where did that come from?", I do know what it is to be a nurse … you look at yourself in the mirror and think "I can do this, I am a nurse", you know I am a good nurse' (Site A NQN13).

(Allan et al. 2016: 383)

In the discussion that follows we consider the transition from being a newly qualified nurse to gaining experience in the practice setting with the support of the preceptor, and in turn your role in developing students of the future. The chapter also includes comments from Zoe at various points, drawing on her very recent experience as a newly qualified mental health nurse receiving preceptorship. This will illustrate and add depth to the points being made and demonstrate the very real and personal experience of becoming a nurse.

We begin the chapter by considering how to effectively use the support that is available. It is possible to be a senior student one day, and the next, on receiving confirmation of successful registration with the NMC, you are a qualified nurse. The enormity of this is immense, and it can be challenging to adapt. In **Chapter 10** we discuss *'impostor phenomena'* which is a response to finally attaining the role for which you have long wished, and an aspect of being able to effectively make the transition to embrace this new identity.

Learning outcomes

- An understanding of preceptorship.
- Learning as a newly qualified nurse, and the Six Senses Framework.
- Supporting students and junior learners, and 360 degree feedback.

In navigating the transition from senior student to newly qualified nurse it is helpful along the way to monitor your thoughts as this process unfolds. To help you in this endeavour this chapter emphasises the process of socialisation in becoming a nurse. This is important, as we want to *'fit in'*, yet at the same time to not do this at the expense of our principles, values and that which we hold in highest regard. While negligent or unsafe practice is clearly dealt with through other formal and legal processes, due to the demands of clinical practice sometimes we encounter working areas where there is a stagnant or inflexible culture. You may not feel empowered at this early stage of your career to initiate change and influence the culture of clinical areas. However, we will consider the Six Senses Framework, and factors which we can develop to improve team-working and morale. These offer practical and feasible measures that in themselves are not profound but promote good team-working and will improve the effectiveness and quality of care.

The final section of this chapter discusses 360 degree feedback and Hawkins and Shohet's (2012) seven-eyed model of clinical supervision. In developing effective role models and nursing supervisors and assessors of the future it is helpful to view the learning–teaching relationship as a 360 degree learning experience. We therefore end the chapter by thinking about the learning experience during pre-registration education in its entirety, so that you see yourself not only where you are now but in the context of your development so far, and what the future holds. Such a perception will help you see your career in nursing in context and encourage self-development while optimising your capacity to effectively reach your potential, and in doing so will represent an inspiring role model for future nursing students.

Some of the points that are made in this chapter might present views about how newly qualified nurses feel which echo experiences and feelings that you already recognise. There is a benefit in this in at least three respects. Often it is possible to believe that the feelings we experience are unique and individual and that can challenge your confidence and self-belief. Discovering that others have felt the same way is reassuring in knowing that you are not alone. Secondly, if some of the issues discussed in this chapter are already familiar to you this means that your development may be well on track, and you are well prepared and ready for the next stage of transition. As a student nurse I remarked to my personal tutor that in being a participant observer of assessments I sometimes felt frustrated at not being able to have greater involvement, as issues were sometimes not being discussed that I felt ought to be covered. The tutor responded that I could regard this as a positive, as this suggested that I was ready to practise autonomously. Finally, it is heartening and offers hope to hear about the success of others in overcoming challenges or simply just success-fully adapting to the responsibility of being a qualified nurse.

PRECEPTORSHIP

Increasingly there is an emphasis on measures to make transition points in nursing more seamless. For example, newly qualified nurses support students learning in practice, so that nurses at all stages of the course, and immediately post-qualification, can develop in a more measured fashion (see **Chapter 3**). Yet very positively, and in the spirit of lifelong learning, this also extends to the important period following qualification in the form of preceptorship.

Preceptorship has long been recommended as a means of orientating newly qualified nurses into their role and was introduced in 1991 with the transition of nurse training from an apprentice-orientated practice-based model to adopting a new theoretical approach (Irwin et al. 2018). The intention was for preceptorship to support newly qualified nurses to make the transition from a basic safe prac-titioner to a competent and confident nurse. Preceptorship provides a structured learning experience, offering formal support in the early stages of post-qualified nursing practice. Generally, newly qualified nurses receive preceptorship for the first year upon commencing their first role (Health Education England [HEE] 2019), with the preceptor being a more experienced nurse who has been qualified for at least twelve months (Quek and Shorey 2018). Most Trusts and health care providers have policies regarding preceptorship, and specific packages that it is a requirement to complete, in order to lend the relationship structure and focus.

The learning methods used in preceptorship vary, ranging from regular individ-ual meetings to study days and structured clinical supervision (Irwin et al. 2018). In their systematic review of the literature Irwin et al. (2018) identified that the literature is equivocal as to the effectiveness of preceptorship in achieving the intended goals of ensuring that preceptees become competent and confident professionals. This is possibly because of ambiguous outcome measures, and a lack of common criteria and methods of assessing the preceptee's progress. However, a systematic review by Edwards et al. (2015) identified that transitional support strategies make a positive impact, irrespective of what they are.

The content of preceptorship is outlined in Table 4.1. There is a focus in precep-torship on roles specific to a practitioner functioning at the level of accountability of a qualified nurse in terms of coordinating and organising care. Yet there is also an emphasis on competence in clinical procedures, and the skills necessary for the practical performance of the role. The nature of these specific tasks will vary depending on the work of the specialist area; however, examples which will apply to many areas include medicine administration, dressing changes, escalating dete-riorating patients, incident reporting, infection control and monitoring vital signs.

Zoe describes this as follows:

Any setting your nursing career starts with will have its own unique team and way of working to get to grips with. I think as long as you are transparent, admit what you don't know and own what you do there is no limit.

This second aspect of preceptorship might involve the preceptor liaising with the newly qualified nurse and the charge nurse or line manager if there are concerns about the preceptee's capability and performance, or further training is needed. The scope of preceptorship is recommended as covering the aspects listed in Table 4.1.

Table 4.1   Aspects of a preceptorship programme

Accountability	Leadership
Career development	Quality improvement and audit
Communication	Medicines management
Conflict management	Resilience and sustainability
Delivering safe care	Reflection and self-awareness
Emotional intelligence	Safe staffing/raising concerns
	Team-working

Source: adapted from HEE, 2019

Together the preceptor and preceptee work through the preceptorship programme. In addition to the more standard aspects of preceptorship and functioning at the level of qualified nurse, Ockerby et al. (2009) draw attention to the individual nature of the relationship and emphasise that preceptorship also focuses on individual needs.

Activity 4.1

Look at the aspects of preceptorship identified in Table 4.1. In relation to each one think of a clinical scenario in which this was an issue. For example, it might be that you were a student on a shift where there was a high level of staff sickness and the team were working below the recommended staffing level. You might find positive examples, as well as negatives. Consider what you would do if you were the nurse in charge for each of these examples.

In their integrative review of the literature Quek and Shorey (2018) identified that the preceptor generally performs this role in addition to their other demanding clinical duties, leading to inconsistencies in the level of support. As a result, and due to preceptorship being less prioritised than direct patient care, the learning needs of the preceptee may not always be met.

In contrast with previous learning during nurse training the preceptor–preceptee relationship is different and less hierarchical, as the preceptor is another staff nurse, and so a peer with the newly qualified nurse and has a different form of relationship with the learner. Preceptorship therefore represents an induction into the nursing community, and a process of socialisation to the reality of being and becoming a qualified nurse.

Imagine you are on your preceptorship as a newly qualified nurse. You are permitted to choose your preceptor.

Think of three characteristics that the preceptor might possess that would be especially useful for you.

Now think about these characteristics. Consider the reason(s) for choosing these specific attributes.

Some people prefer to learn by being challenged or stimulated, while others prefer support and peer-led learning where they can acquire knowledge alongside the person from whom they are learning. Price (2013) discusses 'real-time clinical reasoning' explaining that often when learning students are able to consider decisions related to practice freed from the pressures of time and situation. In qualified practice the nurse is often presented with a dilemma, and expected to make a decision or act. Confronted with this, the newly qualified nurse might confer with their mentor, in what Bott et al. (2011) refer to as a 'five minute preceptor conversation'. Within this, discussion the newly qualified nurse summarises what is happening, yet also the action that is required and presents the rationale(s), or evidence supporting the choice of action. The preceptor then discusses with the preceptee the rules that emerge from the situation, before identifying positives in the preceptee's analysis of the situation and identifying any learning or developmental needs.

Consider what other methods of learning in practice with your preceptor you might be able to identify.

Activity 4.2

The reality of becoming a qualified nurse can present us with experiences and feelings that we could not have anticipated. Working as a newly qualified nurse in any setting will be anxiety provoking. Zoe comments on her first day, and on adopting a professional demeanour:

The first day I was petrified but this had to be internalised, whilst there's always a place for reflection and noticing the feelings you are having, first impressions are also pivotal. Confidence was key, at least definitely acting that way was crucial. The fact is many staff and patients will have seen a number of new nurses over the years, they will know more than you if you are likely to stay. Showing from day one that whilst you and everyone else knows you have a lot to learn, you are capable will go an awful long way. The ability to be assertive with patients from day one and pick up the ward routine quickly is invaluable.

Yet Zoe also felt:

If I had felt too out of my depth or that I could not do it I am sure support would have been available.

When first qualifying I was well aware of my skills and strengths which had been emphasised by the qualified nurses with whom I worked when assessing my performance as a senior student in leading shifts. However, when I began to work as a newly qualified nurse the position reversed, and while no one criticised my performance, I when privately reflecting on my performance I tended to highlight my perceived mistakes and limitations.

In hindsight the stress I experienced was unnecessary, and I was being excessively self-critical. Therefore, it helps to monitor your own thoughts and recognise your own mind-set, and challenge yourself. If you are prone to engaging in self-criticism, it is worth recognising negative automatic thoughts (NATs) and reframing them to create a more positive idea, in order to balance how you view situations (Skinner and Wrycraft, 2014). An example might be after a shift remembering you have forgotten to do something that was handed over; for instance, reordering some medication held in stock in the ward clinic room. The negative automatic (NAT) thought might be: *'I forgot to order the medication; that's another thing I forgot. I always forget something. I'm so stupid!'* The thought might be reframed to become more positive and constructive in terms of self-talk but also helpful in developing your practice.

Activity 4.3

Question: Think of an alternative viewpoint that might offer some balance to my self-critical thought in the above example.

Suggested answer: This is only my suggestion, but an alternative thought might be: *'I forgot to order the medication. That's a shame but I had a lot to remember and it was a really busy shift. Still, there's no point giving myself a hard time about it now, as that will not change things. But in future I can remember how I feel now and next time concentrate as hard as I can so as not to forget anything.'*

This thought has two positive uses. It reduces self-criticism which does not help us perform better and introduces a positive action that can be taken in practice to reduce the potential of the same error occurring. This technique resembles cognitive restructuring which is used in Cognitive Behavioural Therapy (CBT).

It is also sometimes worth appraising our concerns. There are some issues for which there may be significant potential for harm, either immediate, or over time. While we should not become complacent, it is worth considering whether the anxiety that we feel about an issue is proportionate to the actual level and extent of risk. This can be hard to discern, and so may require discussion with the preceptor or another more experienced colleague, but developing this skill will help us to prioritise, know where to direct our attention and allow us to better manage stress during the difficult early days of post-registered practice.

Recognising our *'self-talk'* and where we may be engaging in self-criticism will reduce stress, introduce perspective and help us practise in a more self-aware manner, and ensure that work does not intrude too much into our private leisure time. This will allow for the enjoyment of time off-duty, ensure that we keep up with hobbies, interests and recreational activities, and maintain relationships and enjoy the quality of life which will allow us to renew our energy levels when we are away from work. It is also the case that working in the role that we have trained for so long for may be rewarding.

Zoe remarks:

On my way home I reflected on my experience; it felt a really positive one and I was excited to get back. I felt I had made a good impression on staff and patients.

THE NATURE OF LEARNING AS A NEWLY QUALIFIED NURSE

The qualified nurse is regarded as a competent professional, having successfully passed all of their theory and practice assessments to satisfy all of the stages of pre-registration training. While discussing preceptorship we have looked at the core content and developed an understanding of what we can expect from the preceptor as a source of support. Yet the nature of your learning will be different than when you were in nurse education, and this leads us to consider the nature of learning while on preceptorship.

In professional education Lave and Wenger (1991) have suggested the notion of 'communities of practice' (Wenger 1998; Wenger et al. 2002). Their work refers to a range of different professions, including business, and has been highly influential in professional education, yet was not specifically developed in nursing. Within 'communities of practice' complex issues in a work-based setting are rendered amenable to specific problem-solving solutions that are not derived from formal learning. 'Communities of practice' develop around discrete and specific knowledge which is neither formalised nor codified yet represents the spirit and core of the values that are inherent to the profession. Essentially training within the profession becomes a process of socialisation to a 'community of practice' involving exposure to tacit learning, and the acquisition, interpretation and application of profession-specific knowledge. Critics such as Boud and Middleton (2003) suggest that 'communities of practice' may not provide sufficiently developed frameworks within which to structure learning. However, it may be argued in response to this that 'communities of practice' are by definition adaptable and flexible forms of learning which are not conducive to being harnessed within a formalised approach. Viewed through the lens of this theory, preceptorship can be seen as orientating to the social situation of being a nurse.

This aspect of the role is demonstrated by this comment from Zoe:

> Fitting into the Team was important, particularly the healthcare assistants as they spend the most time looking after the patients. I was worried about this before I started as these types of hospitals are historically institutionalised and I was worried I would not find a place there. I couldn't have been more wrong, the people were kind and helpful and I have received fantastic feedback from the team. My advice here would be get to know your team – they have been my biggest allies particularly in this environment. Be confident to make decisions and delegate tasks but also make a few rounds of tea and coffee. Also, value experience, training has taught you so many skills and our knowledge is up to date and relevant, however, it is important to recognise those who have been there years. That first shift was long, our shifts are 7.30–21.30, however it flew by as has every other shift since. There is also that incredible luxury of 4 days a week off.

In addition to a wide-ranging process of socialisation there are other characteristics specific to the newly qualified nurse's learning needs. It has been noted that newly qualified nurses experience challenges in adopting a leadership role. In their research Ekstrom and Idvall (2015) found that a supportive environment and well-functioning teams encourage newly qualified nurses to take on and embrace a leadership role. In another research study conducted at three hospital sites in the UK between 2011 and 2014 Allan et al. (2016) explored the role of invisible, unplanned and unrecognised learning in newly qualified nurses' delegation of tasks and supervised health care assistants. Their rationale for investigating this phenomenon was that delegation and supervision are commonly regarded as skills that are developed while *on the job'* and represent invisible knowledge. Interestingly Allan et al. (2016) identify that learning occurs in and through the clinical area. It is developed by observing others, coaching and learning alongside peers, but also through ideas and concepts associated with work and from other areas of our experience.

Yet whereas the formal academic content of the curriculum provides struc-tured learning with clear criteria and outcomes, in contrast invisible learning in practice is often triggered by the setting and context. In this situation knowl-edge is re-contextualised and adapted to circumstances which do not fit the norm, and where responses may need to be adapted to a different set of circumstances. In this sense knowledge is fluid, adaptable and has multiple meanings and applications.

However, it has also been identified that in some cases clinical knowledge is evident in established routines, practices and hierarchies, in a form of codified knowledge which is a necessary part of professional practice (Allen et al. 2015; Evans et al. 2010). Therefore, learning to become an experienced nurse involves knowing when to follow established protocols, being able to recognise when to adapt existing knowledge to another use, and knowing when to improvise. This understanding is developed through immersion in clinical practice, and can appear to be invisible knowledge, yet is a tacit and very real process. Allen et al.'s (2016) findings identified invisible learning as occurring in four main areas. These are: learning from mistakes; learning as a result of difficult experience(s); learning through informal instruction from colleagues; and just muddling through.

Duchscher (2008a) identified 'transition shock' and suggested that this can last up to the first four months of qualified practice. Duchscher (2008b) also identifies that during the first year of practice the newly qualified nurse passes through three stages of learning supported by their preceptor. These stages are: doing, knowing and being (Figure 4.1). This represents a growth in certainty and confidence in the role.

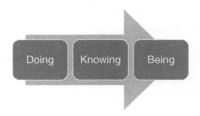

Figure 4.1   Duchscher's (2008b) stages of transition

The transition that the newly qualified nurse undergoes as depicted in Figure 4.1 represents a deepening in learning and understanding. The newly qualified nurse moves from a purely prescriptive role (doing) where we perform a certain range of tasks and functions; to being aware of why we do what we do (knowing); and finally assuming the role, and not having to consciously reflect on why we do what we do. This is synonymous with Knowles' theory of andragogy (see **Chapter 10**). Yet we can also make sense of this using Barbara Proctor's (1987) model of clinical supervision. This model is composed of three aspects, forma-tive, normative and restorative (Table 4.2).

Table 4.2   Proctor's model of clinical supervision

Aspect	Features	Actions
Formative	Education and professional development	Formal training and education
Normative	Carrying out the role	Performing competencies and skills; organising care
Restorative	Coping; how we feel about what we do	

Source: adapted from Proctor, 1987

The formative and normative aspects are important in contributing to how nurses learn and undertake the role. Yet the restorative aspect reaffirms our core purpose and continuing motivation, and links together the formative and normative aspects. As the nurse gains in experience and skills the formative and normative aspects of learning become less of an immediate concern. While there may be changes in legislation or new procedures introduced requiring further training and instruction and revisiting the formative and normative aspects of the model, our predominant focus of learning as we gain experience becomes concerned with the restorative.

An illustration of this notion is that when undergoing the management placement, the student learns how to lead a shift. Often specific functions are performed, such as task delegation, monitoring the performance of work, and the general progress and moving forward of patients' care. The student is assessed in basic skills commensurate with the level of performance that might be expected of a first level nurse. At this point the senior student is engaged in the normative aspect of clinical supervision of Proctor's (1987) model. The reflection and de-brief that they may experience with the qualified nurse supporting them will pertain to their achievement in carrying out the skills and competencies of nursing. However, nurses that have been qualified for many years and are very experienced in their role may at the end of a shift reflect on how they feel about what has happened. The learning that occurs is of a more affective, less task-focused nature. In terms of amount the learning may be less. However, consistent with the notion of time as discussed in **Chapter 3**, as nurses develop they may re-evaluate previous experiences and see new and emergent meanings which were embedded and not obviously apparent at the time.

THE SIX SENSES FRAMEWORK

As a newly qualified nurse it is important to consider your resilience, and how you will ensure sustainability in the role. In **Chapter 2** we discussed finding a job and identifying a role for which you are suitable that will nurture you in the important early days of post-qualified practice. However, sometimes toxic or unhelpful cultures can become embedded in clinical areas which may not be visible to the unacquainted eye until you begin to work there as a qualified nurse. In some cases, it may be that the staff justifiably feel unvalued or unsupported, and are required to cope in situations where there are limited resources yet seemingly infinite demands, or are expected to take responsibility beyond the scope of their role. The enthusiasm and idealism of a newly qualified nurse entering this environment may be resented or unwelcome by tired and disillusioned staff. However, there may be long-term strategies we can adopt in order to slowly develop and foster change and create positive cultures and pockets of safety and responsible practice in situations where staff may feel unsafe, disempowered and disillusioned.

Cooper et al. (2013) carried out an action research project on an inpatient ward to identify how a group of staff for whom 'learned helplessness' and 'socially structured defence techniques' (2013: 1729) impeded their engagement with developing practice. Although the study consisted of just a limited number of thirteen semi-structured interviews, and took place in one clinical area, the findings noted that over time improvements were made with a reduction in the use of defence techniques by the staff. The positive change was attributed to the 'presence and neutrality of the researcher who worked together with staff on their issues of concern' (Cooper et al. 2013: 1729), and the staff being involved in the process of change.

These are obvious and quite simple actions, and it is perhaps worth also investigating the leadership culture that led to a negative environment taking hold to begin with. Nevertheless, at a ward-based level an implication for practice from Cooper et al.'s (2013) research was that staff-centred initiatives offer the potential to create effective and productive nursing teams. A useful framework which has been the focus of the work of several academics and researchers (Andrew et al. 2011; Brown et al. 2008a, 2008b; Nolan et al. 2006; Ryan et al. 2008) is the Six Senses Framework originally developed by Nolan et al. (2006) as a relationship-based approach intended for use in clinical areas delivering care for older inpatients. In your role as a newly qualified nurse the elements of this framework offer the potential to promote a positive culture among staff in clinical settings. Brown et al. (2008b) adapted the Six Senses Framework for use by students. However, in Table 4.3 it has been interpreted to apply to ward-based staff or the members of a clinical team.

Furthermore, there are specific terms and language used in this approach, with the values of the Six Senses Framework regarded as an 'analytical lens' through which we can appreciate whether practice and the delivery of patient care is 'enriched' or 'impoverished' (Brown et al. 2008b). Brown et al. (2008a, 2008b) also suggest that unless staff embrace the values of the Six Senses, they are unlikely to be able to facilitate them for their patients. Often values-based frameworks depend on the authenticity and commitment of the staff entrusted to implement these initiatives to be successful.

Hunter (2010) undertook a small-scale qualitative research study into students' experience of Emergency Department (ED) placements using the Six Senses Framework. Emergency Departments are especially useful placements

Table 4.3   The Six Senses Framework

Sense	Characteristics
Security	Feeling able to develop in professional role and competence, and be supported
Belonging	Feeling included, and valued, and having a role within the team
Continuity	Cohesion between the professed purpose and remit of the clinical area and the care that is being delivered and work of the team
Purpose	Having a focus, and meaningful personal and professional goals
Achievement	Progress and achievement being fairly and proportionately recognised and acknowledged
Significance	Feeling that your contribution to the delivery of care matters and makes a difference

Source: adapted from Brown et al., 2008b

for student nurses, offering the acquisition of a wide range of clinical skills. Rapid socialisation, readily available learning opportunities, and useful feedback and support, which are all factors that are prevalent in the Six Senses Framework, are useful and were remarked upon as helpful in their learning by students participating in Hunter's (2010) research. Therefore, the Six Senses Framework provides a useful set of values which can be used in promoting positive team-working and helping to create positive and open working environments that will engender support, trust and circumstances in which practitioners will feel comfortable. This is clearly desirable for newly qualified nurses, yet these are values which you can espouse in contributing to developing good team-working.

In the next and final section of this chapter we look at 360 degree feedback, and the contribution that this can make to your development and transition towards becoming an experienced nurse.

360 DEGREE FEEDBACK

360 degree feedback is identified as gathering information on a person's performance from a variety of perspectives (Bergman et al. 2014). In their research Hensel et al. (2010) found that this is of more use in an organisation that focuses on personal growth than administration. Bracken et al. (1997) identified that opinions differ as to whether 360 degree feedback ought to be introduced with the rationale of benefiting the whole organisation, or specifically with the intention of developing individuals. Atkins and Wood (2002) conducted research on where there were variations between the self-rating of performance by the individual and the rating of others. Their findings suggest that variations are predicated based on subjective bias. Where performance is being scored or seen as *'good'* or *'bad'* the subjective view of the staff member and the person rating them can influence

performance appraisal above objective assessment. Consistent with Hensel et al. (2010) and Bracken et al. (1997), 360 degree feedback seems to be especially suited to nursing, and especially for those in preceptorship. Seeking feedback from numerous perspectives provides useful information on qualitative aspects of the preceptee's development.

Hawkins and Shohet (2012) developed a comprehensive model of clinical supervision that views situations from multiple perspectives. This links with the notion of 360 degree feedback, by being concerned not only with the supervisee's perspective but those of other people with whom they come into contact during the course of their clinical work. The benefit of Hawkins and Shohets' (2012) model is to deepen nurses' capacity to empathise with the perspective of others with whom they come into contact but also to appreciate the effect that they have on other people, and be able to appraise their own competence and growing confidence.

Furthermore, this cultivates a flexible mind-set in the newly qualified nurse, and a way of looking at situations freed from purely their own perspective, needs and values. Hawkins and Shohet's model refers to practitioners and therapists working in mental health settings. In the interpretation offered in Box 4.1 the model is seen in terms of the nurse and patient. The model may be used in reflective conversations with preceptors or colleagues. It may be that the situation or relationship on which you are reflecting is with a colleague. While many of the stages refer to the nurse–patient relationship and working therapeutically, it is possible to substitute these for working alongside colleagues. So for example, if I am reflecting on delegating a task to a colleague I may still use Eye 1 but interpret this aspect from the perspective of my colleague.

The seven eyes of the model are described in Box 4.1.

Box 4.1   Hawkins and Shohet's (2012) seven-eyed model of supervision

Eye 1: **The focus of the patient**. From this viewpoint the newly qualified nurse seeks to empathise, and see things from the patient's perspective, in terms of what is important to them, and what they value and want from their care.

Eye 2: Interventions. What interventions do we use with the patient? Why do we adopt certain styles of communication, or interact in a particular way with the patient? What do we filter out between what we think and what we say to the patient?

Eye 3: **The nurse–patient relationship**. The therapeutic rapport is the milieu through which we bring about positive change for the patient. However, while we work for the patient's best interests, by its nature nursing involves emotions, and while these have positive elements there are also other less favourable

(Continued)

(Continued)

aspects. At times we might feel guilty, angry or resentful, or patients might expose our vulnerabilities as people and remind us of family members or other people we have known. It is helpful to view this aspect of the model in terms of imagining the patient in another aspect of our life, for example someone we just happened to meet. Removing the relationship from the context of health care permits us to see the patient as a person, and not the pathologised set of features we often perceive.

Eye 4: Focus on the nurse's process. We are privileged in our access to our own inner mental life. However, our feelings can often be elusive and hard to identify. In this aspect of the model, we are asking what we feel about the patient. What do we feel that the patient is communicating to us, for example, feelings of dependence, anxiety and fear about their health, or helplessness?

Eye 5: Nurse–supervisor relationship. Patterns of relationships between the nurse and patient can be replicated in clinical supervision in the relationship between the newly qualified nurse and the clinical supervisor, in a parallel process.

Eye 6: Supervisor's process. This concerns how the supervisor can act as a catalyst in supporting the newly qualified nurse in understanding more about their work with patients. It may also involve the supervisor noticing parallel processes, and ways in which the newly qualified nurse–clinical supervisor relationship may have emotional elements resembling the therapeutic relationship with patients.

Eye 7: The wider context. This takes account of the influence of other organisations with whom the nurse works and other members of the multi-disciplinary team, such as doctors. It includes the influence of the organisation and policies and procedures; the work environment; and the family, relatives and significant others of patients.

Source: adapted from Hawkins and Shohet, 2012

Consistent with the seven-eyed model of supervision, when learning as a newly qualified nurse it is necessary to expand our awareness. As a student nurse we begin by focusing on our personal performance, and then during the latter stages of training, when leading shifts, we begin to expand the scope of our awareness. Understanding the perspective of others, whether this is members of the clinical team, patients, family, relatives, carers and significant others, or aspects of the wider environment means that we will become better at anticipating issues with which we need to deal, and better able to assess and approach problems and to respond to changing circumstances.

Powell (1993) identifies several useful points concerning the nature of change:

- Change is **constant** and **inevitable**;
- Change occurs as a **result of insight** and **differing behaviours** in the **right amount** and at the **right time**;
- Focus on **what can be changed**, as opposed to what cannot.

An additional piece of advice on this theme is that a small change can make a big difference. Through engaging in deep reflection with regard to a wider range of perspectives we will realise and understand more about practice. While it may feel premature, taking every opportunity to work with and support the learning of students and junior staff from the very beginning of your qualified practice will assist with your development. There are several reasons why this is a good idea. Firstly, it is important to continue to learn and keep curiosity alive. Secondly, as a recently qualified nurse you are familiar with the curriculum, and able to understand the needs and perspective of students. Most importantly of all, while teaching and facilitating supervision might feel like an empowered role, often the teacher or clinical supervisor is learning together with the learner. Coaching and teaching involves enjoyment in learning and exercising curiosity, which will extend your knowledge and understanding of practice.

In this chapter we have discussed an understanding of preceptorship in orientating the newly qualified nurse. Preceptorship performs a useful role in easing the transition, and contributing to developing nurses' competence and confidence, yet also in orientating and socialising the new practitioner to the realities of qualified practice. Next, we looked at how newly qualified nurses learn, considering the type of learning, and looking at the Six Senses Framework as a discrete set of positive values that might be cultivated to promote a positive and trusting and transparent culture in clinical areas.

Finally, we discussed 360 degree feedback, and considered Hawkins and Shohet's (2012) seven-eyed model of clinical supervision as a method of deep and wide-ranging reflection to expand your perspective on practice and develop your skills. This chapter ends with Zoe's words, but the point on which we end is the same one with which we began. This comment has been chosen because if in the midst of immense doubts and challenges you feel overwhelmed and unsure of what to do, take a deep breath and then listen to the voice inside you which is calmest and clearest, and that will provide your answer.

Zoe's words:

Nothing can ever fully prepare you for your first day as a qualified nurse; it is the most terrifying and exciting day of your life. University can train you to deal with the transition and your cohort can be invaluable; however, like the autonomy we try and instil in our service users the person responsible for getting you through this transition period is you. Knowing yourself, when to ask for help, being willing to look at new approaches and staying true to the type of nurse you have promised yourself you will be are key.

REFERENCES

Allan, H.T., Magnusson, C., Ball, E., Evans, K., Horton, K., Curtis, K. and Johnson, M. (2015). People, liminal spaces and experience: understanding recontextualisation of knowledge for newly qualified nurses. *Nurse Education Today*, 35: 78–83.

Allan, H.T., Magnusson, C., Evans, K., Ball, E., Westwood, S., Curtis, K., Horton, K. and Johnson, M. (2016). Delegation and supervision of healthcare assistants' work in the daily management of uncertainty and the unexpected in clinical practice: invisible learning among newly qualified nurses. *Nursing Inquiry*, 23: 377–85.

Andrew, N., Robb, Y., Ferguson, D. and Brown, J. (2011). 'Show us you know us': using the Senses Framework to support the professional development of undergraduate nursing students. *Nurse Education in Practice*, 11: 356–9.

Atkins, P.W.B. and Wood, R.E. (2002). Self-versus others' ratings as predictors of assessment center ratings: validation evidence for 360-degree feedback programs. *Personnel Psychology*, 55(4): 871–904.

Bergman, D., Lornudd, C., Sjöberg, L. and Von Thiele Schwarz, U. (2014). Leader personality and 360-degree assessments of leader behaviour. *Scandinavian Journal of Psychology*, 55: 389–97.

Bott, G., Mohide, A.E. and Lawlor, Y. (2011). A clinical teaching technique for nurse preceptors: the five minute preceptor. *Journal of Professional Nursing*, 27(1): 35–42.

Boud, D. and Middleton, H. (2003). Learning from others at work: communities of practice and informal learning. *Journal of Workplace Learning*, 15(5): 194–202.

Bracken, D.W., Dalton, M.A., Jako, R.A., McCauley, C.D. and Pollman, V.A. (1997). Should 360 degree feedback be used for developmental purposes only? Greensboro, NC: Center for Creative Leadership.

Brown, J., Nolan, M. and Davies, S. (2008a). Bringing caring and competence into focus in gerontological nursing: a longitudinal, multi-method study. *International Journal of Nursing Studies*, 45: 654–67.

Brown, J., Nolan, M., Davies, S., Nolan, J. and Keady, J. (2008b). Transforming students' views of gerontological nursing: realising the potential of 'enriched' environments of learning and care – a multi-method longitudinal study. *International Journal of Nursing Studies*, 45: 1214–32.

Cooper, J., Meyer, J. and Holman, C. (2013). Advancing knowledge on practice change: linking facilitation to the senses framework. *Journal of Clinical Nursing*, 22: 1729–37.

Duchscher, J.E.B. (2008a). Transition shock: the initial stage of role adaption for newly graduated registered nurses. *Journal of Advanced Nursing*, 65(5): 1103–13.

Duchscher, J.E.B. (2008b). A process of becoming: the stages of new nursing graduate professional role transition. *Journal of Continuing Education in Nursing*, 39(10): 441–50.

Edwards, D., Hawker, C., Carrier, J. and Rees, C. (2015). A systematic review of the effectiveness of strategies and interventions to improve the transition from student to newly qualified nurse. *International Journal of Nursing Studies*, 52(7): 1254–68

Ekstrom, L. and Idvall, E. (2015). Being a team leader: newly registered nurses relate their experiences. *Journal of Nursing Management*, 23: 75–86.

Evans, K., Guile, D., Harris, J. and Allan, H.T. (2010). Putting knowledge to work: a new approach. *Nurse Education Today*, 30: 245–51.

Hawkins, R. and Shohet, R. (eds) (2012). *Supervision in the Helping Professions*, 4th ed. Maidenhead: Open University/McGraw-Hill.

Health Education England (2019). *Preceptorship and Return to Practice for Nursing*. www.hee.nhs.uk/sites/default/files/documents/preceptorshipframework_booklet%20FINAL.pdf, accessed 21 June 2019.

Hensel, R., Meijers, F., Van der Leeden, R. and Kessels, J. (2010). 360 degree feedback: how many raters are needed for reliable ratings on competency development? *International Journal of Human Resource Management*, 21(15): 2813–30.

Hunter, D. (2010). How clinical practice placements affect professional development. *Emergency Nurse*, 18(5): 30–4.

Irwin, C., Bliss, J. and Poole, K. (2018). Does preceptorship improve confidence and competence in newly qualified nurses? A systematic literature review. *Nurse Education Today*, 60: 35–46.

Lave, J. and Wenger, E. (1991). *Situated Learning: Legitimate Peripheral Participation*. Cambridge: Cambridge University Press.

Nolan, M., Brown, J., Davies, S., Nolan, J. and Keady, J. (2006). *The Senses Framework: Improving Care for Older People Through a Relationship-Centred Approach: Getting Research into Practice (GRIP). Report No. 2*. Sheffield: University of Sheffield.

Ockerby, C.M., Newton, J.M., Cross, W.M. and Jolly, B.C. (2009). A learning partnership: exploring preceptorship through interviews with registered and novice nurses. *Mentoring & Tutoring: Partnership in Learning*, 17(4): 369–85.

Powell, D. (1993). *Clinical Supervision in Alcohol and Drug Abuse Counseling*. San Francisco: Jossey-Bass.

Price, B. (2013). Successful preceptorship of newly qualified nurses. *Nursing Standard*, 28(14): 51–6.

Proctor, B. (1987). Supervision: a cooperative exercise. In M. Marken and M. Payne (eds), *Enabling and Ensuring Supervision in Practice*. Leicester: Youth Bureau and Council for Education and Training in Youth and Community Work.

Quek, G.J.H. and Shorey, S. (2018). Perceptions, experiences, and needs of nursing preceptors and their preceptees on preceptorship: an integrative review. *Journal of Professional Nursing*, 34: 417–28.

Ryan, T., Nolan, M., Reid, D. and Enderby, P. (2008). Using the Senses Framework to achieve relationship-centred dementia care services: a case example. *Dementia*, 7(1): 71–93.

Skinner, V. and Wrycraft, N. (2014). *CBT Fundamentals: Theory and Cases*. Maidenhead: Open University Press/McGraw-Hill.

Wenger, E. (1998). *Communities of Practice: Learning, Meaning and Identity*, 6th ed. Cambridge: Cambridge University Press.

Wenger, E., McDermott, R. and Snyder, W. (2002). *A Guide to Managing Knowledge: Cultivating Communities of Practice*. Boston, MA: Harvard Business School Press.

PART II
During the transition process

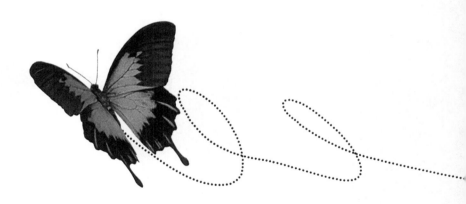

5

Ethical and legal aspects of care

Patricia Macnamara

'Bevan, who had fought hard to get his plan through Attlee's post-war Labour cabinet, was determined the NHS should "universalise the best" care and not simply act as a safety net for the poor, and should be based on need, rather than ability to pay.'

(Denis Campbell, 2016)

As nurses we are entrusted with the care of our fellow humans when they are often at their most vulnerable and this means we incur great responsibility and accountability. This chapter will look at the basis for that moral responsibility and how this in turn has led to the development of the legal and regulatory mechanisms which have been developed to protect the safety and wellbeing of our patients and clients. When you work in a health care setting you are frequently in situations requiring a moral and or ethical decision, and this requires you to function within legal frameworks and applying legal principles. This chapter highlights the ethical and legal aspects related to professional practice as a nurse. The areas covered will include legislation relating to practice, such as anti-discriminatory legislation and law related to management of care.

Learning outcomes

- Discuss some of the ethical theories which have influenced health care.
- Have a critical understanding of health and social care law and ethics in relation to generic aspects, e.g. consent, confidentiality, duty to care and human rights.

- Understand how these principles have shaped the legal framework of care in England and Wales.
- Critically analyse the application of ethics to patient care and how it relates to health and the rights, duties and responsibilities of professional nurse practice.
- Review of the care or service delivery to individuals and their families with respite and palliative care needs.

There will be an analysis of the statutory provision driving practice coupled with an exploration of current ethical issues, such as resourcing, safeguarding and judicial review, and issues of consent, death and dying, and respecting life. The application of principles, theories and the legislative framework will be presented to you with reflective activities, enabling you to access knowledge, trace the implications, refine the outcomes and evaluate the degree of moral justification you may need to possess.

Ethics discusses how humans should live in order to have the sort of life that enables them to flourish. In the UK we live and work within the western cultural tradition that traces its roots back to ancient Athens where Aristotle (1976) said that the basis for these discussions rested on the fact that humans were social beings who were capable of reason (Barnes, 1979). Aristotle also saw ethics as a practical subject not as a theoretical exercise. In other words, we think about what we should do and then try to do it both as individuals and as a society. This emphasis on the practical is seen in the way we organise society by means of economics, politics and law. It is also shown in the professional codes that have been developed over the last century, an example being the NMC Code (2018).

ETHICAL THEORIES

One of the most influential theories about how society should be organised in order to bring about the greatest benefit for all its members is utilitarianism. A utilitarian bases his/her decisions on the belief that all humans have equal worth and value. Jeremy Bentham (1748–1832) is the name most closely associated with utilitarianism. He believed that 'Nature has placed mankind under the governance of two sovereign masters, pain and pleasure. It is for them alone to point out what we ought to do, as well as to determine what we shall do' (Bentham 2005). This was what determined right and wrong and thus he defined ethics as: 'the production of the greatest possible quantity of happiness' (Bentham 2005).

Utilitarianism is called a consequentialist moral theory because the moral worth of an action is judged by the outcomes, or consequences, that it produces. A utilitarian, according to Bentham, should aim to bring about the 'greatest good for the greatest number'. Bentham also believed that all human beings were equal and as such each person's happiness was of equal importance.

These ideas influenced the development of British democracy throughout the nineteenth and twentieth centuries. The founding of the National Health Service in 1948 can be seen as part of a culmination of this view that the state should view all citizens as equal members of society with equal access to services on the basis of need.

The unit is very busy, and one patient and their family are being very disruptive and noisy. However, they have just received devastating news. How do you both support them and the rest of the ward alongside supporting other staff on the ward?

Activity 5.1

The founding of NICE in 1999 continued this ethical tradition. NICE was originally set up as the National Institute for Clinical Excellence, a special health authority, to reduce variation in the availability and quality of NHS treatments and care. Its name changed to the National Institute for Health and Clinical Excellence in 2005 (NICE 2019) The aim of NICE is to try to achieve the best use of resources available to the health service in order to ensure the best treatment for as many patients as possible across the entire country. The NICE charter states that its aim is to help health, public health and social care professionals deliver the best possible care based on the best available evidence (NICE 2013). One of the main objections to Bentham's formulation of producing the greatest good for the greatest number is the question of what happens to the individual if they are not part of the greatest number and is it ever acceptable to sacrifice individuals for the sake of the common good?

A solution to this problem was provided by John Stuart Mill (1806–73) who was a friend of Bentham and a fellow utilitarian. Mill declared the only purpose for which power can be rightfully exercised over any member of a civilised community, against his will, is to prevent harm to others (Mill 2003). Mill said that individuals should be free to make their own decisions and the only acceptable constraint on that freedom is the harm that may befall others. The ability to make and execute one's own decisions is what is meant by autonomy.

A patient that you are caring for refuses to adhere to the prescribed regime; they have an infection which is highly contagious which could lead to further infections. They argue that it stops them from having a full life because it takes up so much time. How do you work in partnership with them to ensure their decisions are respected and/or acknowledged and they and the general public also remain safe?

Activity 5.2

Health protection legislation in England gives public authorities powers and duties to prevent and control risks to human health from infection or contamination, including by chemicals and radiation.

(Notifiable diseases and causative organisms: how to report, April 2019)

The action of intervening in the apparently autonomous choices of an individual is justified by a utilitarian by the prevention of foreseen harm to others. However, the outcomes of actions cannot always be accurately predicted, either for individuals or for society and thus it has been argued that making decisions based on their outcomes is not a satisfactory foundation for ethical thinking. Rather, it is better to have rules which will be implemented to avoid trying to work out the consequences of a particular action.

MORAL ACTION

The name most usually associated with this approach is that of the German philosopher Immanuel Kant (1724–1804). Kant believed that the basis of moral action was duty and hence this school of ethical thought is described as duty based (Kant 2007). This then gives rise to the question of how it is to be decided that something is a duty and must therefore be carried out?

Kant described three criteria to be considered when trying to determine a rule that must be obeyed:

1. Principle of humanity.
    (a) All humans are members of what he called a kingdom of ends. This means that everyone has their own ends or goals in life, and these must be respected by everyone else.
    (b) A human being can never be just a means to an end.
2. Principle of impartiality.
    This means that all humans have the same standing and that no individual or group of people should be favoured or disadvantaged in relation to another.
3. Principle of universality.
    A moral duty must be universally binding, i.e. it applies in all places at all times without exception.

The NHS Constitution (2013: 3) says: 'The NHS provides a comprehensive service, available to all irrespective of gender, race, disability, age, sexual orientation, religion, belief, gender reassignment, pregnancy and maternity or marital or civil partnership status.' This binds the NHS and all health care professionals to treating all patients impartially.

If all three principles highlighted above are met, then the rule would be a categorical imperative, meaning it must be obeyed by all no matter the circumstances.

This is why a categorical imperative has never been established, because there will always be an exception to the rule. It also fails to consider cultural differences. Most people whether nurse, health professional or member of the public accept that taking another human life is wrong but can think of exceptions to that rule, e.g. in defence of self or others. There is also a problem if there is a conflict between two or more principles, e.g. where telling the truth would mean breaking a confidence. This is especially difficult when dealing with safeguarding issues with vulnerable individuals. It is even more a challenge when dealing with children and young people. A duty-based ethic does not tell us how to resolve this conflict. Its main influence can be seen in approaches to research involving human subjects.

There are a number of relevant legal cases which will be discussed throughout the chapter (see Table 5.1).

Table 5.1 Medical legal cases

Medical legal case	Rationale
Aintree University Hospitals NHS Foundation Trust v James [2013] UKSC 67	In best interest for medical treatment
Bolam v Friern Hospital Management Committee [1957] 1 WLR 582	Appropriate standard of reasonable care in negligence cases involving skilled professionals
Montgomery v Lanarkshire Health Board [2015] UKSC 11	The matter of informed consent
Re C [1994] 1 All ER 819	Adult, refusal of treatment
Gillick v West Norfolk and Wisbech Health Authority [1986]	The matter of age of consent
University College London Hospitals v KG [2018] EWCOP 29	In the matter of the Mental Capacity Act 2005

DIVERSITY AND HOLISTIC CARE

Diversity refers to the differing experiences of all people, individuals and groups, and within the context of health care it has the added dimension of acknowledging these differences within the health care setting. In a study looking at nurses' attitudes to transcultural care, Festini et al. (2009) found that effective communication was the most important aspect of providing culturally competent care. These aspirations fit with the value of safeguarding people which embody anti-discriminatory practice, partnership, and equal opportunities for every citizen. Staff concerned with safeguarding vulnerable individuals are among those in the front line faced with the consequences of the failure of social inclusion measures and the raised expectations of families in need (Bilham 2013). Holistic care is commonly accepted as treating or caring for the person as a 'whole' or 'complete' person and not in terms of a distinct diagnosis or 'part'. There are many cultural implications of this point of view; it is important that all aspects of a patient's background are taken into consideration. This is really what is at the heart of holistic assessment and holistic care.

Activity 5.3

Marilyn Potter is 87 and lives alone in the community. You visit her every day to administer her insulin. She is registered blind and has limited mobility. One morning Marilyn tells you that she is convinced that Gladys, her carer, has been taking money from her purse.

What safeguarding issues does this raise?

What might your initial response be?

Whom should you inform?

Duty of Care: The 'duty of care' refers to the obligations placed on people to act towards others in a certain way, in accordance with certain standards. The term is sometimes used to cover both **professional** duties that health care practitioners may have towards others, but there are distinctions between the two. Generally, the law imposes a duty of care on a health care practitioner in situations where it is 'reasonably foreseeable' that the practitioner might cause harm to patients through their actions or omissions. This is the case regardless of whether that practitioner is a nurse, midwife, health care assistant or assistant practitioner. It exists when the practitioner has assumed some sort of responsibility for the patient's care. This can be basic personal care or a complex procedure.

(Royal College of Nursing, *Duty of care*, April 2019)

Duty of care also needs to be observed for research which is essential to allow new treatments to be developed and care improved, but humans must never be seen simply as a means to obtaining that knowledge. Where possible, research subjects must be willing and knowledgeable participants in trials with the right to withdraw at any time. When this is not possible, e.g. because prospective participants have dementia, then the study must consider their best interests before enrolling them in the proposed study. The application of principles has also influenced the development of policies both nationally and locally as a way of giving safe and effective care.

THE FOUR PRINCIPLES OF BIOMEDICAL ETHICS

The application of principles to health care practice is a useful means of helping us to focus on the patient and can be helpful in avoiding self-interest. The Four Principles approach of Beauchamp and Childress (2013) has become well known as a tool to help health care professionals in making decisions. The principles to be considered are autonomy, beneficence, non-maleficence and justice.

Autonomy: As already mentioned, this means that people who have the ability to make decisions should have these decisions respected. The NHS Constitution (2013: 8) states:

> You have the right to accept or refuse treatment that is offered to you, and not to be given any physical examination or treatment unless you have given valid consent. If you do not have the capacity to do so, consent must be obtained from a person legally able to act on your behalf, or the treatment must be in your best interests.

This acknowledges the autonomy of adults (someone over the age of 18) and thus their right to accept or to refuse treatment that is offered, even when the refusal will lead to death or disability.

Beneficence: As health care professionals you are committed to doing good, and this is what beneficence, the second principle, means. So, although a patient has the right to refuse treatment our legal, ethical and professional duty is to ensure that the decision is freely made by someone who understands the possible or actual consequences of the decision. Similarly, if individuals cannot make their own decision then others must do so for them. The requirement that the health care professionals act in people's best interests if they cannot make their own decisions, e.g. because of dementia, recognises the principle of beneficence.

Non-maleficence: This means that if we as nurses cannot actively do good then we should avoid making things worse, e.g. patients should not acquire new infections as a result of being admitted to hospital. It also means that as a health care professional you have to know and acknowledge the limits of your own competence in order to avoid inflicting harm. This also shows respect for the wellbeing of the patient. An example of failing to recognise one's limitations is illustrated by the case of Violeta Aylward who was a registered Learning Disability nurse. In 2009 she accepted a bank shift which involved caring for a ventilated patient. Ms Aylward acknowledged that she was totally unfamiliar with the skills necessary to look after such a patient. She was filmed accidently disconnecting the ventilator and in the 10 minutes it took to reconnect it the patient suffered catastrophic and irreversible brain damage. She was not prosecuted but was removed from the register by the NMC (2012).

In some instances, e.g. the treatment of Creutzfeldt-Jakob disease, there is no tested treatment available and, in this case, the death rate is 100 per cent within two to three years of diagnosis (NHS 2018). The administration of a new and untested treatment for this condition is dealt with by the Code of Practice to the Mental Capacity Act 2005. At paragraph 6.18, it says: 'Some treatment decisions are so serious that the court has to make them.' Under these circumstances the court has said it is acceptable to use untested forms of medical treatment as things could not be made worse than they already are. In this case the patient was able to contribute to the decision and expressed his willingness to try the new treatment and was supported in this by his family (*University College London Hospital v KG* [2018])

Justice: This means that patients should be treated fairly and equally when considering the distribution of resources and about who gets what when decisions about treatment are made. The establishment of Clinical Commissioning Groups (CCGs) following the Health and Social Care Act (2012) has meant that decisions about the provision of care are made locally. This sometimes means that some resources such as the provision of infertility services vary from one area to another in a National Health Service. As resources are always limited there will always need to be decisions made about treatments offered, but perhaps there should be more public discussion of how resources are distributed.

Thus far we have looked at some of the tools developed to help us as health care professionals make ethical decisions. A common theme that has emerged from all these tools is that all human beings are of equal worth and standing. This arises from an individual's status as a human being and does not rely on anything else. This should be reflected in how we behave towards each other. Professionally the NMC (2018) sets standards for nurses as further discussed in **Chapters 3 and 6** and the NHS Constitution (2013) tells patients and professionals the standards they should expect. The Constitution appeared in 2013 largely in response to the findings of the Francis Report. This had been commissioned because: 'Between 2005 and 2008 conditions of appalling care were able to flourish in the main hospital serving the people of Stafford and its surrounding area' (Francis Report 2013: 7).

The NHS Constitution (2013) sets out rights for patients, public and staff. It outlines NHS commitments to patients and staff, and the responsibilities that the public, patients and staff owe to one another to ensure that the NHS works fairly and effectively. Patients are told in section 3a that: 'You **have the right** to be treated with dignity and respect, in accordance with your human rights'. As already discussed, one of the most important ways of ensuring that the humanity of patients is recognised and acknowledged, and they are treated with dignity and respect is through the right to say yes or no to any treatment offered.

This tells us that the right to make one's own decisions and the idea of determining and acting upon a patient's best interests are seen as vital in order to provide respectful care which upholds the dignity of all patients whether they have capacity or not. In order to ensure that patients are safe, the Health and Social Care Act (2008) established the Care Quality Commission (CQC) in 2009 as an independent regulator of health and social care in England. Their stated aim is to make sure that hospitals, care homes, dental and general practices and other social care services in England, 'provide people with safe, effective, compassionate, high-quality care and we encourage care services to improve' (CQC, 2019).

As well as registering and inspecting services the CQC acts to protect people who use the services, particularly those deemed to be vulnerable as a result of their frailties whether physical, mental or as a result of learning disabilities (see Table 5.2). As a result of the abuse suffered by e.g. residents at Winterbourne View, an assessment centre for people with learning difficulties, in 2011, and Ash Court, a residential nursing home for the elderly, in 2012, the Care Act (2014) establishes the legal framework for safeguarding vulnerable adults in England (NHS 2017b). This is the responsibility not only of institutions but also of individual members of staff.

> All staff within health services have a responsibility for the safety and well-being of patients and colleagues. Living a life that is free from harm and abuse is a fundamental human right and an essential requirement for health and well-being. Safeguarding adults is about the safety and well-being of all patients but providing additional measures for those least able to protect themselves from harm or abuse. Safeguarding adults is a fundamental part of patient safety and wellbeing and the outcomes expected of the NHS. Safeguarding adults is also integral to complying with legislation, regulations and delivering cost effective care.
>
> (The Care Act 2014, ch. 3)

Following the link cited in the reference list to the above will enable you to follow the extensive guidance provided by NHS England in fulfilling your responsibilities as a nurse to your patients.

Table 5.2   Rights issues for individual and mental capacity

Lack of Knowledge	Lack of knowledge and implementation of legal rights for individuals to control their own medical treatment.
	A general lack of rights to self-determination.
Discrimination	Discrimination against individuals on grounds of disability, race, culture, colour, language, religion, gender, and sexuality which can lead to categorisation as mentally ill and subsequent intervention and detention.
Unlawful restriction of liberty	Unnecessary and in some cases unlawful restriction of liberty and inadequate safeguards in mental health and other legislation for individuals.
Inadequate assessment	Inadequate assessment and corresponding lack of care, treatment and education in the criminal justice system.
Use of drugs for containment	Use of drugs rather than for treatment purposes in the community, hospitals, schools, and in other institutions, combined with a lack of knowledge of consent procedures.

(Continued)

Table 5.2   (Continued)

Placement of individuals	Placement of individuals on inappropriate wards in psychiatric hospitals or inappropriate general wards, prison or in other ways detained.
Lack of clear ethical guidelines	Lack of clear ethical guidelines for extreme situations such as force-feedings in cases of anorexia, care of suicide risk, and care of HIV positive or AIDS patients.

Source: adapted from Thurston, 2013

MENTAL CAPACITY ACT 2005

One of the main requirements is the use of the Mental Capacity Act (MCA) (2005). This now governs the law of consent for adults (applies to people aged 16 and over) in England and Wales.

It is based on five principles:

1.   Every adult has the right to make his or her own decisions and must be assumed to have capacity to make them unless it is proved otherwise.
2.   A person must be given all practicable help before anyone treats them as not being able to make their own decisions.
3.   Just because an individual makes what might be seen as an unwise decision, they should not be treated as lacking capacity to make that decision.
4.   Anything done or any decision made on behalf of a person who lacks capacity must be done in their best interests.
5.   Anything done for or on behalf of a person who lacks capacity should be the least restrictive of their basic rights and freedoms.

In English law an adult is anyone over 18 years old and must be assumed to have capacity to make decisions about themselves. If there is any doubt about an adult's mental capacity, then the following questions need to be resolved.

Is there an impairment of or disturbance in the functioning of a person's mind or brain? Examples of impairment could be a learning disability, dementia or permanent brain injury. Disturbances in the functioning of the mind or brain can arise from low oxygen levels, low blood sugar levels in a diabetic, being under the influence of certain drugs, e.g. opiates, both prescribed and recreational and being drunk. A disturbance can usually be corrected but impairment cannot. If it is decided that there is an impairment or disturbance, then the health care professionals need to consider the following:

Is the impairment or disturbance sufficient that the person lacks the capacity to make a particular decision? This means that a person has to have the capacity to make a particular decision and the level of capacity needed will depend upon the seriousness of the decision that needs to be made. Someone may therefore be able to make decisions about what they would like to eat but not about whether or not to have an operation. This also means that because some individuals lack full capacity their rights to make choices and decisions about their lives cannot be ignored or over-ridden. The reason that capacity is so important is because we are asking someone to make a decision about their care or treatment. In order to decide, information is needed and the person must:

Understand the information given to them:
- This is not about language, rather the comprehension of the medical knowledge given.

Retain that information long enough to be able to make the decision:
- This is having the ability to remember all the medical information together long enough to explore all the possibilities.

Weigh up the information available to make the decision:
- Finally, after exploring all the possibilities being able to make a health care decision that the individual is comfortable with.

The question of what information and how much should be given is not easily answered. The Supreme Court's decision in *Montgomery* (2015) established that a health care professional:

> ... is therefore under a duty to take reasonable care to ensure that the patient is aware of any material risks involved in any recommended treatment, and of any reasonable alternative or variant treatments. The test of materiality is whether, in the circumstances of the particular case, a reasonable person in the patient's position would be likely to attach significance to the risk, or the doctor is or should reasonably be aware that the particular patient would be likely to attach significance to it.
>
> (Supreme Court's Decision in *Montgomery* 2015: 11)

The Supreme Court emphasised that whether a risk is material cannot be reduced to percentages, and instead is based on a variety of factors such as:

- Nature of the risk
- Effect on the life of the patient
- The importance to the patient of the benefits of the treatment
- Any possible alternatives
- The risk of those alternatives

The interprofessional team, doctors and you as a nurse need to ensure that any information is provided in a way can be understood by the patient, as required by the MCA (2005), such that the patient understands the seriousness of his/her condition, the benefits and risks and any alternatives so that she/he is able to make an informed decision.

CONSENT

The social markers of adulthood deserve some thought in regard to informed consent, especially related to children and young people in the health care system. It is well commented upon that a person in the UK can drive a car at 17 years but must wait until he or she is 18 years old to purchase alcohol or vote. These different age limits reflect a social judgement about when a person is sufficiently adult to carry out these activities either safely or with sufficient 'adult' judgement. The legal age of consent to sexual activity is set at 16 years because it reflects the social judgement of when a person is sufficiently mature to assume the risks and challenges of sexual activity. However, these social judgements change according to time and geography, and according to other social factors.

Ages of progression to adulthood within UK law:

- **Legally have heterosexual /homosexual sex**: In Great Britain a person has to be 16 or older to have homosexual (gay) or heterosexual (straight) sex.
- **Legally have the right to work full time**: If no longer at school 16- or 17-year- olds are referred to in the law as 'young workers'. Because they are no longer at school, there are fewer restrictions on when they can work and for how long, but there are still some rules.
- **Legally have the right to get married**: In the UK, generally a man and a woman may marry if they are both over 16 and not married or in a civil partnership with someone else. Individuals aged 16 or 17 in England, Wales and Northern Ireland, however, can only marry if they obtain their parents' consent.
- **Legally have the right to live alone**: At 16, young people have the right to decide where they want to live. Some options include: continuing to live at home with their parents or carers, applying for sheltered housing through the council or housing association.

(Adapted from Walker, 2013)

Consent for treatment when children are under the age of 16

Children in this age group are not deemed to be automatically legally competent to give consent. The courts have determined that such children can be legally competent if they have 'sufficient understanding and maturity to enable them to understand fully what is proposed'. This concept is now known as 'Gillick competency' and initially arose in the case of Gillick vs West Norfolk and Wisbech Health Authority in 1986. The term 'Fraser competency' is also used in this respect (Lord Fraser was the judge who ruled on the case).

(Walker 2013: 415)

Consent for treatment when children are aged 16 and 17

Once children reach the age of 16, they are presumed in law to be competent. In many respects they should be treated as adults and can give consent for their own surgical and medical treatment. The Department of Health recommends that it is nevertheless good practice to encourage children of this age to involve their families in decisions about their care, unless it would not be in their interests to do so. If a competent child requests that confidentiality be maintained, this should be respected unless the doctor considers that failing to disclose information would result in significant harm to the child. A child aged 16–18 cannot refuse treatment if it has been agreed by a person with parental responsibility or the Court and it is in their best interests. Therefore, they do not have the same status as adults.

(Walker 2013: 415)

This gives us as the health care professionals the responsibility of determining what matters to the patient and their family when giving information, in other words a one-size-fits-all explanation will not do, some individuals may need an interpreter, others may need understanding into their religious or culture beliefs. Recognition of this principle is reflected in the GMC's (2008) guidelines on consent. These state that no single approach to treatment or care will suit every patient or apply in all circumstances. Individual patients may want more or less information.

The guidance goes on to state that the amount of information shared with patients will depend on the individual patient and what they want or need to know. Some patients want to know as much as possible while others find that the more they learn the less able they feel to make a decision and therefore prefer to leave matters to you with your nursing knowledge and judgement. Assumptions should not be made about a patient's understanding of risk or the importance they attach to different outcomes. These guidelines are currently under review and the final guidance should be available by the end of 2019. Although they are drawn up for doctors, the Supreme Court in *Montgomery* 2015 has endorsed their patient-focused approach to obtaining consent as a model of good practice. This means that this approach can usefully be adopted by nurses and all other health care professionals.

Having made a decision, the patient must then be able to communicate what this is. This could be by talking, using sign language or even simple muscle movements such as blinking an eye or squeezing a hand. From this it can be seen that gaining consent from a patient is very important. The principles supplied by parliament do not mention consent forms. This is because the emphasis is on consent rather than the means by which it is recorded. A consent form is a means to an end, i.e. it should show that consent has been obtained. In ordinary situations, e.g. providing a wash or giving medication, a verbal discussion followed by one of the options mentioned above has always been considered an adequate means of agreeing to what is proposed.

You have been caring for Mary Murphy who is 30 years old; she has come in to have a hysterectomy due to ongoing pain and bleeding. She has signed the consent form and has now changed her mind. She is a practising Roman Catholic and has concerns that the surgery goes against her religious beliefs.

What would you prioritise to ensure Mary is listened to and supported, while she is kept safe?

Consent forms for operations and other invasive procedures can help to remind all parties of what needs to be discussed and provide evidence of what has been agreed and by whom, e.g. the patient and you as the nurse caring for the patient and the interprofessional team. They are not however usually a legal requirement. If a patient cannot sign a consent form but can give valid consent, then the procedure can go ahead. Parents also sign for their children. It would be advisable for everyone involved to make detailed records of the discussions held and the decisions reached. The quality of the information provided, and the patient's un-coerced agreement are what make consent valid, not a signature on a form. Patients also have the right to change their minds at any point before the anaesthetic, if used, takes effect.

Alan Brown is a patient on your ward. He is 60 years old and has an ulcer on his left leg secondary to diabetes. He also has a diagnosis of schizophrenia. Unfortunately, his ulcer has not responded to treatment and the medical team feel that a below knee amputation is necessary to avoid sepsis. Alan denies that he has diabetes or an infection and does not want the operation. He also says 'I don't want to die. I'm only 60'.

Who should make the decision about Alan's care?
What are his rights under the MCA 2005?

This tells us that respect for patients' autonomy is paramount if a patient has capacity. This includes the autonomy of patients who make decisions that others might consider to be unwise, as we have seen from section 1(3) of the Mental Capacity Act 2005. The assumption is that if treatment is suggested it must be because it is considered to be in the patient's best interests, or it would not have been offered. However, patients may, and sometimes do, have a different understanding of their best interests to that of the professionals. An example of this arose in 1994 when a patient in Broadmoor with a diagnosis of paranoid schizophrenia refused an amputation which he was told was necessary to save his life. The patient accepted that this was the doctors' view, but he disagreed and refused treatment. The judge held that he was competent, i.e. he had capacity. He understood the information he had been given and the possible consequences of his refusal but was able to reach his own decision in opposition to professional advice. A patient cannot be held to lack capacity because they do not agree with the professionals or because they make a decision that others consider to be irrational (*Re C* (Adult, refusal of treatment) [1994] 1 All ER 819).

While the Mental Capacity Act (2005) lays great stress on the importance of respecting and upholding the rights of patients with capacity to make their own decisions, it also recognises in sections 1(5) and (6) that not all adults have capacity and that health care decisions sometimes have to be made on patients' behalf. There are several mechanisms by which this can be done lawfully. The most important of these is an advance decision. To be lawful this has to be valid and applicable. Validity means that it was drawn up by a person over the age of 18 who had capacity at the time of making it.

Applicability means that it applies to the treatment needed at the time it comes into use (section 26(1) Mental Capacity Act (2005)). Some patients have already written Living Wills or an Advance Healthcare Directive; this is seen as legally binding and the person who has undertaken this process can be specific about what medical interventions or action can or cannot be taken if they are incapacitated (www.nhs.uk/conditions/end-of-life-care/advance-decision-to-refuse-treatment/, accessed April 2019)

An advance decision only comes into force when a patient has lost capacity. It can only be used to refuse treatment, e.g. to refuse ventilation, but not to demand it. However, if decisions are being made about treatment it will be a factor to consider if a patient has said that they would want a particular treatment. If the decision states that the patient refuses lifesaving treatment then it must be in writing, signed and witnessed (section 25, Mental Capacity Act (2005)). It is not possible to ask for anything unlawful, e.g. a lethal injection. One of the most important issues to be considered when devising an advance decision is the difficulty of predicting the future. An individual may have seen members of the family suffering from cancer and draw up a directive accordingly but then suffer from a stroke. It is also difficult to predict what advances in the medical treatment of a disease will be made and thus what the prognosis will be. If a patient has an advance decision it is useful if you help to ensure it is reviewed regularly in the light of any developments so that it is a true reflection of the patient's wishes.

LASTING POWER OF ATTORNEY

If there is no advance health care decision, then the next most important means of determining a patient's wishes is through someone who has a Lasting Power of Attorney. This is set up by someone, known as the donor, who is over the age of 18 and while they have capacity. There are two types of Lasting Power of Attorney:

- Health and Welfare
- Property and Financial Affairs

An individual can make one or both. The person or persons given the Lasting Power of Attorney are attorney(s). The donor chooses their attorney(s), who can be anyone they want, and fills in the forms. These can be obtained from the Office of the Public Guardian online or through the post. They must be signed by the donor and witnessed and then registered with the Office of the Public Guardian. Unless the forms are registered, the attorney has no legal standing when decisions have to be made. Registration takes eight to ten weeks according to the government website (Office of the Public Guardian 2017).

The sort of decisions that someone with a health and welfare Lasting Power of Attorney can make include:

- The donor's daily routine (e.g. washing, dressing, eating)
- Medical care
- Moving into a care home
- Life-sustaining treatment

It can only be used when the donor is unable to make their own decisions. You will therefore need to check that the attorney is registered with the Office of the Public Guardian as relatives may not understand the need for this. If there is more than one attorney, then the forms will stipulate if each attorney can act individually or if they must make decisions jointly. A person with capacity may also *end* a Lasting Power of Attorney and you need to check as this must also be registered with the Office of the Public Guardian and the attorney(s) informed.

If a patient who lacks capacity has no advance directive or someone with a Lasting Power of Attorney, a Deputy of the Court of Protection may make decisions on the patient's behalf. This will be someone, usually family or a close friend, who has applied to the court to be made a deputy in order to act as a health and social welfare deputy on behalf of an individual who does not have capacity and where there is no other provision made. Again, you need to have written confirmation of this before confirming agreement with their actions. Remember you always need to put the patient's needs above family and friends and, therefore, if you are not sure seek further advice, either from the clinical area and interprofessional team, your service manager or the Trust's solicitors if required.

If none of the above is in place, then it is the responsibility of you as the health care professional to act in the patient's best interests when deciding on any care or treatment to be given. The Mental Capacity Act (2005) gives some guidance on the factors which should be considered when trying to work out what is in a patient's best interests. In determining what is in a patient's best interests, the person making the determination must consider, so far as is reasonably ascertainable, the following factors, as set out in section 4(6) of the Mental Capacity Act (2005):

(a) the person's past and present wishes and feelings (and, in particular, any relevant written statement made by him when he had capacity).
(b) the beliefs and values that would be likely to influence his decision if he had capacity, and,
(c) the other factors that he would be likely to consider if he were able to do so.

The wording of the Mental Capacity Act (2005) means that while an individual's wishes, etc. need to be considered this does not mean that they will necessarily determine what happens to the patient. The doctor will have the final say about what constitutes best interests unless the courts intervene. In terms of the courts' approach to best interests, Baroness Hale in *Aintree v James* (2013) said:

> in considering the best interests of this particular patient at this particular time, decision-makers must look at his welfare in the widest sense, not just medical but social and psychological; they must consider the nature of the medical treatment in question, what it involves and its prospects of success; they must consider what the outcome of that treatment for the patient is likely to be; they must try and put themselves in the places of the individual patient and ask what his attitude to the treatment is or would be likely to be; and they must consult others who are looking after him or interested in his welfare, in particular for their view of what his attitude would be.
>
> (Aintree University Hospitals NHS Foundation Trust (Respondent)
> v James (Appellant), 2013)

This tells us that the patient's welfare must be considered from all perspectives and not simply that of physical survival. There is also the need to consult those looking after the patient and this of course includes the nurses involved as well as family, friends and other carers. If applying the above all sounds rather daunting then remember there is one simple principle which will meet your ethical, professional and legal responsibilities, that is you must know what you are doing and why. It is also important to remember that we are in the business of health care to make things better (Gawande 2007). If the wellbeing of your patient remains your primary objective, then this will be achieved. To find out more about the issues discussed in this chapter and the wider field of law and ethics as they apply to health care and nurses' working lives it is worth following up the references.

RECOGNITION OF END OF LIFE

It is important for you as the nurse to have made some of the difficult end of life decisions beforehand with the family, but also important to have parallel planning in place, where care prepares for the worst, but hopes for the best. This is especially important as there is considerable unpredictability of disease trajectory for many patients, especially children and young people. The difficulty in accurately predicting death means families often face many acute life-threatening events thinking each one is a terminal event. This is unsurprisingly emotionally and physically exhausting for them. There could also be reluctance on the part of both relatives and professionals to use certain drugs which often become necessary at the end of life for fear of 'causing death' (Clarke 2013).

An essential step in *end of life care* is recognising that the person has probably reached the end of their life, and then acknowledging that for everyone involved with the person, both family and the interprofessional team. Some discussions should take place if possible when the person is in relatively good health, in preparing practically for acute, distressing symptoms and making realistic but flexible end of life and advance care plans (Clarke 2013; NHS 2017a). A decision needs to be made about emergency treatment options and resuscitation, and if necessary, a personalised Resuscitation Plan set out and documented for use by ambulance crews, A&E departments and Primary Care Services (DH 2005). The end of life care plan may include an Advance Care Plan (ACP) which may include decisions regarding withdrawal of treatment and Do Not Attempt Resuscitation (DNACPR) decisions (ACT 2009; DH 2005).

End of life care

When people have made the decision to stop all treatment or when interventions are no longer an option then the hospice services may step in and provide palliative care for individuals with life-limiting conditions and their families for as long as it is needed. Care is delivered by a multi-disciplinary team and in partnership with other agencies; hospice services take a holistic and flexible approach to care, and are shaped by the physical, emotional, social and spiritual needs of both the individual and their family. There are currently over 200 adult and 44 children's hospices in the UK providing a range of services within purpose-built centres as well as providing hospice care at home. The services offered by hospices are extensive and are delivered in a variety of environments which includes the home and hospices (Clarke 2013). Some hospices may focus on the person who is terminally ill, while others, especially for children and young people, offer services to individuals with life-limiting conditions, many of which have been present since birth and are now affecting the person's quality of life.

The importance of the culture, religion and spirituality aspects of the hospice movement is that they provide a context in which people can make sense of their lives, explain and cope with their experiences and find and maintain a sense of hope and peacefulness during end of life care. While not all writers agree on the benefits of religion within an end of life context, there remains evidence that religious spirituality can have clear benefits in terms of coping with illness and the threat of death.

The principles of end of life care services for children are broadly the same as for adults. Communication with family and professionals (both verbal and written is crucial to effective end of life care (ACT 2004; DH 2008). Good end of life care requires good teamwork and planning. The 'Gold Standards Framework' for end of life care in adults in the UK details three steps (identify, assess, plan) and emphasises the importance of communication, coordination and control of symptoms (Corr and Balk 2010). These principles work just as well in children's palliative care.

You will need to carefully consider and manage care of the individual and the family at the time surrounding and after death as this can have an emotional impact on the family's memories. Well-managed and well-supported end of life care is a key component of palliative care services. It is impossible to overestimate the extent to which the level and type of care provided can affect the family's experience of the loss of their family member (Clarke 2013).

REFERENCES

Aintree University Hospitals NHS Foundation Trust (Respondent) v James (Appellant), (2013) www.supremecourt.uk/cases/docs/uksc-2013-0134-judgment.pdf, accessed August 2019.

Aristotle (1976). *The Nicomachean Ethics*. London: Penguin.

Association for Children with Life-Threatening or Terminal Conditions (ACT) (2003). The Royal College of Paediatrics and Child Health (RCPCH). *A Guide to the Development of Children's Paediatric Services*, 2nd ed. Bristol: ACT.

Association for Children with Life-Threatening or Terminal Conditions (ACT) (2004). *A Framework for the Development of Integrated Multi-agency Care Pathways for Children with Life-Threatening and Life-Limiting Conditions*. Bristol: ACT.

Association for Children with Life-Threatening or Terminal Conditions (ACT) (2009a). Children's Hospice UK. *Right People, Right Place, Right Time*. Bristol: ACT.

Association for Children with Life-Threatening or Terminal Conditions (ACT) (2009b). Children's Hospice UK. *Making the Case for Children's Palliative Care*. Bristol: ACT.

Barnes, J.A. (1979). *Who Should Know What? Social Science, Privacy, and Ethics*. London: Penguin Books.

Beauchamp, T. and Childress, J. (2013). *Principles of Biomedical Ethics*, 7th ed. Oxford: Oxford University Press.

Bentham, J. (2005). *An Introduction to the Principles of Morals and Legislation*. New York: Prometheus Books.

Bilham, S. (2013). Cultural aspects for children and young people. In C. Thurston (ed.), *Essential Nursing Care for Children and Young People: Theory, Policy and Practice*. London: Routledge, pp. 81–96.

Campbell, D. (2016) 'Nye Bevan's dream: a history of the NHS', *The Guardian*, 18 January, www.theguardian.com/society/2016/jan/18/nye-bevan-history-of-nhs-national-health-service.

Care Act (2014). www.gov.uk/government/publications/care-act-2014-part-1-factsheets.

Care Quality Commission (2019). *About Us*. www.cqc.org.uk/about-us.

Clarke, S. (2013). Children and young people with life-limiting conditions. In C. Thurston (ed.), *Essential Nursing Care for Children and Young People: Theory, Policy and Practice*. London: Routledge, pp. 318–60.

Corr, C. and Balk, D. (2010). Children's Encounters with Death, Bereavement, and Coping. New York: Springer.

Department of Health (DH) (2005). *Commissioning Children's and Young People's Palliative Care Services*. Every Child Matters: Change for Children.

Department of Health (DH) (2008). *Better Care, Better Lives: Improving Outcomes and Experiences for Children, Young People and their Families Living with Life-Limiting and Life-Threatening Conditions*. London: HMSO.

Festini, F., Focardi, S., Bisogni, S., Mannini, C. and Neri, S. (2009). Providing transcultural nursing to children and parents: an exploratory study from Italy. *Journal of Nursing Scholarship*, 41(2): 220–7.

Francis, R. (2013). *Report of the Mid Staffordshire NHS Foundation Trust Public Enquiry*. www.gov.uk/government/publications/report-of-the-mid-staffordshire-nhs-foundation-trust-public-inquiry.

Gawande, A. (2007). *Better*. London: Profile Books.

General Medical Council (2008). *Consent: Patients and Doctors Making Decisions Together*. www.gmc-uk.org/ethical-guidance/ethical-guidance-for-doctors/consent.

Health and Social Care Act (2008). www.legislation.gov.uk/ukpga/2008/14/pdfs/ukpga_20080014_en.pdf.

Kant, I. (2007). *Critique of Practical Reason*. London: Penguin.

Mental Capacity Act (2005). www.legislation.gov.uk/ukpga/2005/9/pdfs/ukpga_20050009_en.pdf.

Mental Capacity Act Code of Practice (2016). www.gov.uk/government/publications/mental-capacity-act-code-of-practice.

Mill, J.S. (2003). *On Liberty*. New York: Dover Publications.

National Institute for Health and Care Excellence Annual Report and Accounts 2017/18, Her Majesty's Stationery Office.

National Institute for Health and Care Excellence (NICE) (2013). www.nice.org.uk/Guidance/MPG2, accessed August 2019.

National Institute for Health and Care Excellence (NICE) (2019). www.nice.org.uk/guidance, accessed August 2019.

NHS (2017a). *End of Life Care*. www.nhs.uk/conditions/end-of-life-care/advance-decision-to-refuse-treatment/.

NHS (2017b). *Safeguarding Adults*. www.england.nhs.uk/wp-content/uploads/2017/02/adult-pocket-guide.pdf.

NHS (2018). *Creutzfeldt-Jakob Disease*. www.nhs.uk/conditions/creutzfeldt-jakob-disease-cjd/.

NHS Constitution (2013). www.nhs.uk/choiceintheNHS/Rightsandpledges/NHSConstitution/Pages/Overview.aspx.

Nursing and Midwifery Council (NMC) (2012). *Fitness to Practice Outcomes*. www.nmc.org.uk/globalassets/sitedocuments/ftpoutcomes/2012/march/reasons-aylward-cccsh-20120315.pdf.

Nursing and Midwifery Council (NMC) (2018). *The Code:* Professional Standards of Practice and Behaviour for Nurses, Midwives and Nursing Associates. www.nmc.org.uk/standards/code/.

Notifiable diseases: causative agents report for 2019 (2019). www.gov.uk/government/publications/notifiable-diseases-causative-agents-report-for-2019, accessed September 2019.

Office of the Public Guardian (2017). www.gov.uk/government/organisations/office-of-the-public-guardian.

RCN (February 2019). *Duty of Care*. www.rcn.org.uk/get-help/rcn-advice/duty-of-care.

Thurston, C. (ed.) (2013). Essential Nursing Care for Children and Young People: Theory, Policy and Practice. London: Routledge.

Walker, S. (2013). The challenges of sexual exploration for young people. In C. Thurston (ed.), *Essential Nursing Care for Children and Young People: Theory, Policy and Practice*. London: Routledge, pp. 257–75.

6

Responsibilities regarding fitness to practice

Chris Thurston and Marty Chambers

'Competence assessment was now a fundamental aspect of pre-registration nurse training with practice learning defined in curriculum development, but the practice assessment of students was the responsibility of the mentor whose role would be to produce a student fit for practice at the end of the educational course.'

(Cassidy, 2009: 39)

The focus of the chapter will be to outline the principles of transitioning from Fitness for Practice (FfP) to Fitness to Practice (FtP) and to explore the understanding of processes used for both student education and qualified nurses when fitness to practice is being questioned. The NMC set the standards that must be maintained by student nurses, as well as the standards that you must meet as you enter and stay on the register. Pre-registration nursing standards include specific guidance for each of the four pre-registration nursing specialisms: Adult, Children's, Learning Disabilities and Mental Health; these changed in 2019 to further enhance the protection of the public. One of the main changes is to split the role of the mentor into assessing and supporting. The role of mentor will disappear, and the students will have a supervisor in practice and a separate practice assessor. You may support the students alongside the supervisor as a coach to begin with and then, after learning the different roles of supervision and assessment, have students of your own.

Learning outcomes

- The role of the NMC in relation to fitness to practice.
- Practise effectively always within your own boundaries of competence, from student nurse, during transition and beyond.
- Act immediately if you believe that there is a risk to patient safety or public protection.

The NMC (2009b) in the code for student nurses reminded you that your conduct is important in upholding the reputation of the profession, both when you are studying and in your personal life. The competency framework from the NMC (2014) set out the standards for competence that every nursing student must acquire before applying to be registered at the first level on the nurses' part of the register. There are separate sets of competency requirements for each of the four fields of adult nursing, mental health nursing, learning disabilities nursing or children's nursing. Each set is laid out under the following four domains.

1. Professional values

    All nurses must act first and foremost to care for and safeguard the public. They must practise autonomously and be responsible and accountable for safe, compassionate, person-centred, evidence-based nursing that respects and maintains dignity and human rights.

    (NMC 2014)

2. Communication and interpersonal skills

    All nurses must use excellent communication and interpersonal skills. Their communications must always be safe, effective, compassionate and respectful. They must communicate effectively using a wide range of strategies and interventions including the effective use of communication technologies. Where people have a disability, nurses must be able to work with service users and others to obtain the information needed to make reasonable adjustments that promote optimum health and enable equal access to services.

    (NMC 2014)

3. Nursing practice and decision-making

    All nurses must also meet more complex and coexisting needs for people in their own nursing field of practice, in any setting including hospital, community and at home. All practice should be informed by the best available evidence and comply with local and national guidelines. Decision-making must be shared with service users, carers, families and informed by critical analysis of a full range of possible interventions, including the use of up-to-date technology.

(NMC 2014)

4. Leadership, management and team working

All nurses must be professionally accountable and use clinical governance processes to maintain and improve nursing practice and standards of healthcare. They must be able to respond autonomously and confidently to planned and uncertain situations, managing themselves and others effectively. They must create and maximise opportunities to improve services. They must also demonstrate the potential to develop further management and leadership skills during their period of preceptorship and beyond.

(NMC 2014)

Each domain was comprised of a generic standard for competence and a field standard for competence. It also includes the generic competencies that all nurses must achieve and the competencies to be achieved in each specific field. The number of field competencies varies in number in each domain and between nursing fields of practice (NMC 2014).

All pre-registration nursing programmes included standards for students to care for all patient groups. It is important that all registered nurses can deal with most nursing roles. Effective from 31 March 2015, and revised September 2018 to include nursing associates, the NMC Code reflects the world in which nurses live and work today, and the changing roles and expectations of nurses. It is structured around four themes: *prioritise people, practise effectively, preserve safety* and *promote professionalism and trust* (NMC 2018a). This chapter will reinforce that care should be person-centred.

A code for students within the UK appeared in 2009 when *Guidance on Professional Conduct for Nursing and Midwifery Students* was introduced by the NMC following awareness that the public could not always see the difference between students and qualified nurses (NMC 2009b). An example of how these status challenges may have affected you as students was cited by Ousey and Gallagher (2007), who reported that students have often been asked to 'lift' a patient even though they are taught at university to 'move' patients using the appropriate manual handling techniques and equipment. The discord of the theory–practice gap may not simply be attributed to a disparity in knowledge by qualified nurses; however, the practices of nurses that influenced you as students, either by their secondary role of undertaking your summative assessment or because of unsafe traditions on the ward, are difficult to change. Therefore, you may have been discouraged from using the recommended techniques in practice. As you transition through to qualification you need to remember these challenges and support students who may also be facing these difficulties.

A research project based on a self-report questionnaire gave a number of reasons for the inappropriate lifting of patients, citing 'lack of equipment', difficulty of 'saying no diplomatically' and 'lack of time' (Ousey and Gallagher 2007). The overall findings suggested that bringing about changes in practice requires action on several levels. Whether teaching in classrooms or on wards or placements, there can be a professional disassociation where nurses, especially student nurses, feel disempowered. This may have caused you and other students to experience ethical dilemmas in practice, and difficulty in deciding when to say no to poor practice.

On placements your learning was assessed by predetermined competency-based objectives in the form of clinical outcomes in practice documents against which you were assessed and supported in your learning by your practice mentor, now to be supervisor and/or assessor. In the final year of your course there are typically only minimum levels of supervision, and an expectation of you performing to a high level of accountability consistent with evidence-based practice, with your conduct consistent with a practitioner that is about to become a registered nurse. At this stage you should have been practising at a level of proficiency and accountability, creating learning experiences and opportunities for yourself and others (Stuart 2007). The skill-based curriculum which has formed the template for your learning on the pre-registration nursing course incorporates current nursing theory and vital aspects of technical competence together with an emphasis on providing person-centred care to develop nurses whose skills reflect the variety and range of capabilities for contemporary practice. Yet consistent with the continual and rapid pace of change in health care the Nursing and Midwifery Council (NMC) has issued new guidance on standards for competence for pre-registration education in 2019.

Increasingly there has been debate nationally and internationally regarding how nursing education programmes protect the public (MacLaren et al. 2016). It has been suggested that the university has responsibility for the monitoring of the FfP of pre-registration students during their programme, while the practice area has responsibility for the practical aspects of 'on the job' training. The National Nursing Research Unit (NNRU 2009) suggests that there are varying understandings of competence and a disparity between the university-based perception of competence and that in practice. On the one hand, in practice competence is reductionist and depends upon whether the student nurse is capable in the performance of tasks, while academically at university, competence is seen as the ability to link practice-based knowledge and theoretical critical thinking.

Goudreau et al. (2009) suggest that competency is based on you being able to mobilise knowledge, skills, attitudes and external resources and then applying them appropriately to situations. Scott Tilley (2008) concluded that competency standards must be achieved for entry onto the register, but evidence is required of collaboration between education and service providers. This suggests that whilst power is transferred to your mentors or supervisors/assessors, the weight of accountability and responsibility in terms of passing or failing students can be confused by the differing agendas between your chosen university and your current clinical setting. Even so, by supporting you in the learning environment, the mentor, supervisors/assessors evaluate competency and appraise your needs to achieve satisfactory standards of proficiency, and must be considered key to ensuring FfP.

As a third-year student nurse you reach the competent level of skills acquisition which are best taught by demonstration and case studies offered by the proficient or expert-level practitioners you work alongside. Ritualistic practice within nursing has been replaced by evidence-based care and a new educational approach adopted, but as nurses we still struggle to learn from each other. An aspect of this is when nurse assessors are unable to fail students, and important professional judgements of character and clinical skills may not be being made properly.

Gainsbury (2010) discussed a survey of nearly 2,000 nurse mentors and found that 37 per cent indicated that they have passed students whose competencies or attitude concerned them, or whom they felt they should have failed. The survey found that these decisions were due to being unable to substantiate their concerns, while 31 per cent believed the university would overturn a fail (Gainsbury 2010). The profession cannot be assured of a truly reflexive mentor/supervisor to demonstrate FfP if practice and university do not have open dialogue about students' competence. Hunt et al. (2016) also confirmed that mentors often feel emotionally manipulated by failing students; while this is not common, it is a challenge and may lead to mentors/supervisors refusing to have students. If you have challenges in your placements, how will you ensure this does not occur for the students you support? This may include ensuring you receive further support as you take on the role and having discussions with the relevant nurse tutor for the student.

According to Cassidy (2009) effective practice-based learning occurs when situated in a holistic context of care, involving patients' experiences and aided by reflexive and inclusive mentors/supervisors. Furthermore, as a result, 'responsive assessment' can be the basis for a reciprocal student–mentor relationship, and by fostering this partnership model, learning and assessment strengthens the connections between formal theory underpinning practice and the informal acquisition of clinical knowledge. However, Freshwater and Stickley (2004) suggest that the lack of clarity regarding the concept of emotional intelligence can affect the qualified nurse's belief systems to identify the assessment and competency of those practical skills demonstrated by the student nurse. This must be matched with a 'holistic assessment' inclusive of the process of enquiry between student and mentor (Cassidy 2009: 41).

FITNESS FOR PRACTICE

Being Fit for Practice (FfP) required you as a student nurse to develop the skills, knowledge, good health and good character by the end of your course to do your job safely and effectively. One study aimed to evaluate FfP definitions within pre-registration programmes in Scotland to determine whether students achieve FfP by the end of their course (Holland et al. 2010). Using a mixed methodology of three phases involving questionnaires, Objective Structured Clinical Examinations (OSCE), curriculum evaluation, semi-structured interviews and focus groups, four distinct themes were established. The first theme defined FfP as the acquisition of skills, knowledge and attitudes. The authors suggested that 'someone who is not fit to practice is not fit for practice' but no one distinct definition could be concluded (Holland et al. 2010: 463). The remaining themes referred to preparation for practice, being in practice and partnerships in practice.

Mentoring and/or supervising is the influence, direction and guidance which can be provided by a close, experienced and trusted counsellor. Mentorship and/or supervising in nursing helps student nurses and health care staff to develop through support and positive role modelling competencies, self-confidence, networking, socialising and career opportunities for the student being supported (Huybrecht et al. 2011). The important element of this is role modelling of competency and evidence-based practice which has the patient or client in the centre of any care or decision-making process.

Activity 6.1

Looking at the themes highlighted above, reflect on the specific elements which are required for either third-year students, or when you qualify. Examples are given to get you started (Table 6.1).

Table 6.1   Examples for Activity 6.1

Theme	Specific elements for third year	When qualified
Skills knowledge and attitudes	Example:	Example:
	Medicine management for your group of patients with support from your mentor	Administering intravenous medication
Preparation for practice	Example:	Example:
	Arranging the skill mix required for the patients in your care	Managing the duty roster
Being in practice	Example:	Example:
	Using evidence-based patient care	Ensuring all members of the team undertake evidence-based practice
Partnerships in practice	Example:	Example:
	Work cooperatively as a member of the interprofessional team	To work within and lead both nursing and interprofessional team as required

Woodcock (2009) reminds all nurses that if the student's practice is assessed as still being unsafe, it is the mentor's/assessor's professional and legal responsibility to fail them. Furthermore, the attribution of 'caring' balances the knowledge, skills and attitudes necessary for effective nursing care, which must compel the mentor/assessor to move from a check-list scenario (for example giving an injection) to a comprehensive understanding of the behavioural processes nurses apply. From 1 January 2009 the recommendation from the NMC was for all course providers to establish local 'Fitness' processes and panels to consider any health or character issues regarding students, to ensure that public protection is maintained. This promotes the smooth transition of student placements alongside the acquisition of academic insights, allowing nursing courses to embody the application of theory to practice direct to the training of students in patient care.

a. Reflect upon a situation either in practice or in university where you raised concerns, and this was handled positively.

What was the outcome?

b. Reflect upon a situation either in practice or in university where you raised concerns, and this was handled inadequately.

What was the outcome?

c. Reflect upon the difference: why was one positive and the other not so?

Think about:

The two different situations

The different individuals involved including who led the interaction

The ability of different individuals to actively listen

The ability of individuals to admit their mistakes and to take responsibility for their action and its impact

Activity 6.2

The NMC had previously produced mandatory standards identifying the responsibility and accountability of mentors/assessors, but a final year mentor/assessor had also to ensure that the student met additional criteria to be able to make the final judgement about whether the student has achieved the overall standards of competence required for entry to the register (NMC 2008). However, the NMC requires further confirmation at the end of each course that both practice and theory parts have been successfully achieved in partnership with the university as the awarding body (NMC 2008). Moving forward from 2019, the NMC requires all qualified staff to support students, such as occurs in midwifery and, alongside this, the Nominated Academic Assessor makes a final decision as to whether the student has been successful in theory while the Nominated Practice Assessor does the same for practice.

As a student you needed mentors or supervisors in practice to facilitate your learning and the assessment process and ensure the quality of your learning experience through development and innovation. The mentor (supervisor or coach) is: 'the nurse, midwife or health visor who facilitates learning and supervises and assesses students in the practice setting' (Bray and Nettleton 2007: 849). Therefore, the assessment of your practice as a student was the responsibility of your mentor or more recently your assessor. In order for you to be considered fit for practice, the assessment approach should have been vigorous and highlighted your strengths, investigated concerns and identified that you were being supported and managed both academically and professionally (Reid 2010).

Yet consistent with the continual and rapid pace of change in health care, the NMC has issued new guidance on standards for competence for pre-registration education, starting in 2019 and in place across the country by 2020.

The NMC comment:

The changing nature of the health and care environment and the ways services are delivered is having a significant impact on registered nurses' practice. The future context of nursing practice is being challenged by economic, social and political factors including changes in skill mix, the increase in unregistered support workers and proposals to create a new nursing support role. These challenges provoke questions into what the future registered nurse will look like and how pre-registration education will need to be structured in the future to equip newly qualified nurses with the scientific, technical and professional skills needed for practice.

(CoDH/NMC Roundtable: The Future Focus of
Nursing Education, March 2016)

While your course involved an equal emphasis on theory and practice, the increased emphasis on the academic currency from the university has led at times to technical evidence and skill replacing caring, and education supplanting nursing as a vocation. However, working together, the clinical trusts and the universities are promoting an awareness of the importance of teamworking, commitment to the development of positive working relationships, and the cultivation of active skills in team building and working necessary to produce a nurse fit for practice. You have undertaken throughout your course competence assessments which are now a fundamental aspect of pre-registration nurse training, with practice learning and the responsibility of your qualified mentor, supervisor and practice assessment handled more recently by the practice assessor (Cassidy 2009: 39).

Registered nurses were responsible for the assessment of your practice in the clinical setting and academic tutors did so when you were in the university setting; this approach is now evolving as the NMC has revisited which qualified professionals undertake your summative assessment. This relationship requires a different approach to the management of professional conduct and performance. The RCN and the NMC recommend curriculum adaptions and standard setting within the three-year course, while nurse education has re-evaluated its assessment of competency to ensure that learning outcomes and specific skills are identified.

From 2019 the NMC, after revisiting the requirements of nurse pre-registration education by discussing the challenges with patients, nurses and employers, has developed key components of the roles, responsibilities and accountabilities of registered nurses. This includes the expectations of the student when transitioning to newly qualified status; the requirements of the learning environment are also explored to ensure a safe and enhanced learning experience.

> We believe that this approach provides clarity to the public and the professions about the core knowledge and skills that they can expect every registered nurse to demonstrate. These proficiencies will provide new graduates into the profession with the knowledge and skills they need at the point of registration which they will build upon as they gain experience in practice and fulfil their professional responsibility to continuously update their knowledge and skills.

> (NMC 2018b: 3)

There are seven performance platforms (see Table 3.1) offered by the NMC to plan safe nurse education to become FfP and to have ongoing competency and conduct to remain FtP.

PLATFORM 1

Being an accountable professional

> Registered nurses act in the best interests of people, putting them first and providing nursing care that is person-centred, safe and compassionate. They act professionally at all times and use their knowledge and experience to make evidence-based decisions about care. They communicate effectively, are role models for others, and are accountable for their actions. Registered nurses continually reflect on their practice and keep abreast of new and emerging developments in nursing, health and care.

> (NMC 2018b: 7)

Reflect on this performance platform. How has your role as an accountable professional changed since you have qualified as compared to being a student?

Activity 6.3

This first platform makes it clear that from the start of a nursing course, as students you needed to be aware of your actions, and that as you qualify and support students you need to ensure you practise positive role modelling – this includes keeping up to date with evidence-based clinical care. It also includes continuing to reflect on your practice and undertake Continuous Professional Development (CPD) related to your area of practice. Fitness to practice is also about conduct; there is a need to behave compassionately with all individuals involved, even in the most difficult situations.

PLATFORM 2

Promoting health and preventing ill health

Registered nurses play a key role in improving and maintaining the mental, physical and behavioural health and well-being of people, families, communities and populations. They support and enable people at all stages of life and in all care settings to make informed choices about how to manage health challenges in order to maximise their quality of life and improve health outcomes. They are actively involved in the prevention of and protection against disease and ill health and engage in public health, community development and global health agendas, and in the reduction of health inequalities.

(NMC 2018b: 10)

Activity 6.4

Reflect on this performance platform. How has your role in promoting health and preventing ill health changed since you have qualified as compared to being a student?

Platform 2 is about both student nurses' and qualified nurses' role in health promotion. This needs to work in several ways – at a personal level by not smoking, being of a healthy weight and moderate in terms of drinking as an important start. Also, you need to report any illness you have which may affect your ability to practise in a competent manor. Finally, while formalised health promotion is very important, often it is opportunistic education which may have the greatest impact; for example, on an acute admission to hospital giving a mother who smokes opportunistic education and support for cessation programmes when their child has asthma, highlighting the clear benefits from giving up smoking. This should be approached in a sensitive manner with offers of appropriate support.

PLATFORM 3

Assessing needs and planning care

Registered nurses prioritise the needs of people when assessing and reviewing their mental, physical, cognitive, behavioural, social and spiritual needs. They use information obtained during assessments to identify the priorities and requirements for person-centred and evidence-based nursing interventions and support. They work in partnership with people to develop person-centred care plans that take into account their circumstances, characteristics and preferences.

(NMC 2018b: 13)

Reflect on this performance platform. How has your role in assessing needs and planning care changed since you have qualified as compared to being a student?

Activity 6.5

Platform 3 acknowledges the need to work in partnership with the patient and their families from initial assessment through to the conclusion of their care. Some patients may have beliefs and lifestyles that may be very different from your own. It is a professional requirement to respect these, if they are not detrimental to others. A simple example may be religious food requirements; more complicated may be the withdrawal of treatment, or the right to die agenda. If you do not feel confident or professionally competent to deal with the situation senior practitioners should be contacted for support and further guidance. If this is not available or not forthcoming, contact senior management; again, if no support is offered, you may need to seek outside professional support.

PLATFORM 4

Providing and evaluating care

Registered nurses take the lead in providing evidence-based, compassionate and safe nursing interventions. They ensure that care they provide and delegate is person-centred and of a consistently high standard. They support people of all ages in a range of care settings. They work in partnership with people, families and carers to evaluate whether care is effective, and the goals of care have been met in line with their wishes, preferences and desired outcomes.

(NMC 2018b: 16)

Reflect on this performance platform. How has your role in providing and evaluating care changed since you have qualified as compared to being a student?

Platform 4 highlights the requirement to ensure that when working in clinical practice you are up to date on the status of your patients. It is unacceptable professional conduct to assume that the assessment and actions undertaken in the morning are still appropriate in the afternoon without a review. This can be dangerous in acute settings, where a patient's condition can change minute to minute, especially following interventions such as surgery. Evaluation should be a continuous cyclical activity and, following the evaluation, changes in intervention should be made if required. When clinical situations are not so acute, it is still a priority regarding patients and clients. The multi-professional team need to decide the frequency of the evaluation required; this review of care needs to have a holistic approach.

PLATFORM 5

Leading and managing nursing care and working in teams

Registered nurses provide leadership by acting as a role model for best practice in the delivery of nursing care. They are responsible for managing nursing care and are accountable for the appropriate delegation and supervision of care provided by others in the team including lay carers. They play an active and equal role in the interdisciplinary team, collaborating and communicating effectively with a range of colleagues.

(NMC 2018b: 19)

Reflect on this performance platform. How has your role in leading and managing nursing care and working in teams changed since you have qualified as compared to being a student?

Platform 5 requires an examination of how senior students and qualified nurses need to lead teams of carers. When you oversee a team, you need to work with other colleagues' strengths and challenges. Junior staff will copy both professional practice and incompetent or unprofessional practice. This includes how you are collaborating with other professionals; this can be a difficult situation at times; however, as an advocate for both patients and staff, it is important to remain open to communication in a flexible and professional way. Working with and leading your team in a professional manner regardless of the clinical area will ensure a high standard of care. An example may relate to the care given on the older persons' ward, where you encourage all team members, both nursing and other members of the multi-professional team, to optimise the ward environment by ensuring every interaction has a social element. This should include a clear introduction of who they are as a professional and their name and what intervention they would like to do. However, to enhance this further, both verbal and nonverbal communication should be comfortable for the older person, especially if there are challenges to mental health such as dementia.

PLATFORM 6

Improving safety and quality of care

Registered nurses make a key contribution to the continuous monitoring and quality improvement of care and treatment in order to enhance health outcomes and people's experience of nursing and related care. They assess risks to safety or experience and take appropriate action to manage those, putting the best interests, needs and preferences of people first.

(NMC 2018b: 21)

Reflect on this performance platform. How has the role of improving safety and quality of care changed since you have qualified as compared to being a student?

Activity 6.8

Platform 6 reminds all nurses that unless unrealistic or mortally dangerous, patients' needs and wants should be the priority. This can be a challenge with budget and resource constraints; however, creative ideas for care if risk assessed and of a good quality can be just as cost effective as traditional approaches. An example of this has been different coloured disposable medication pots for different prescription times, especially useful for patients who take their medication with food. The patients would not be obligated to take their tablet on an empty stomach or with an unwanted snack. The coloured pots are no more expensive than the white pots and ensure easy monitoring of patients taking their medication. This approach supports both patients' wishes, and safe quality of nursing care.

PLATFORM 7

Coordinating care

Registered nurses play a leadership role in coordinating and managing the complex nursing and integrated care needs of people at any stage of their lives, across a range of organisations and settings. They contribute to processes of organisational change through an awareness of local and national policies.

(NMC 2018b: 24)

Activity 6.9

Reflect on this performance platform. How has your role in coordinating care changed since you qualified compared to when you were a student?

Platform 7 acknowledges that when coordinating care, at clinical, hospital or organisational level it is important to evolve practice, with the insights from research and evidence-based practice. While some traditional practice has stood the test of time such as regular medication and meal times, other traditions have been shown to cause damage such as people with learning disabilities being kept in institutions rather than living in the community. Strong forward-looking leadership enables patient-centred care to be the first thought when changing and evolving care.

Moving forward from 2019, the NMC has suggested it is better to separate the role of supervision in practice, to permit more objective assessment of clinical competence. This change followed an NMC consultation, which found that named mentors did not always have the time to support students. Therefore, it is an expectation that all nurses and midwives should become supervisors or coaches. In the past there has been confusion over the difference between the role of mentor and sign-off mentor, a lack of institutional support for the mentorship role, and a failure of mentors to manage failing students. Therefore, when supporting and assessing students, all registrants should be responsible for the supervision of students, and supervision and assessment are separate undertakings. This will include you in your role of newly qualified nurse. The NMC will also no longer prescribe standards on the training of supervisors and assessors. Instead there will be freedom for organisations to develop their own models, to allow for local circumstances, and utilise the skills of staff that are already experienced mentors.

The NMC's *Realising Professionalism: Standards for Education and Training Part 2: Standards for Student Supervision and Assessment* (2018c), explores how student nurses' learning needs to be undertaken.

Effective practice learning

All students are provided with safe, effective and inclusive learning experiences. Each learning environment has the governance and resources needed to deliver education and training. Students actively participate in their own education, learning from a range of people across a variety of settings.

(NMC 2018c: 5)

All students have the right to a safe learning environment which has been audited, and support from both clinical educators and university educators.

Supervision of students

Practice supervision enables students to learn and safely achieve proficiency and autonomy in their professional role. All NMC registered nurses, midwives and nursing associates are capable of supervising students, serving as role models for safe and effective practice.

(NMC 2018c: 6)

All qualified staff, which includes you right after qualification to the register, have a requirement to support and supervise students; this enables the enhancement of nursing students' learning environment. Also, it acknowledges that learning occurs anywhere that students encounter patients, clients and their families. When a student's competency or conduct is in question it is important to have discussions with all professionals who have worked with the student; this will include you in your role as their support.

Assessment of students and confirmation of proficiency

Student assessments are evidence based, robust and objective. Assessments and confirmation of proficiency are based on an understanding of student achievements across theory and practice. Assessments and confirmation of proficiency are timely, providing assurance of student achievements and competence.

(NMC 2018c: 8)

All assessors need to balance the role of supporting students during the assessment process with the priority to protect the public. Students need direction and support through the clinical placement; however, if concerns are raised by you or any other professional it is everyone's responsibility to bring this to the attention of the assessor.

The NMC go on to highlight the roles in the clinical area in supporting and assessing students (see **Chapter 3** for more details).

Practice supervisors: role and responsibilities

Practice supervisors serve as role models for safe and effective practice in line with their code of conduct. Support learning in line with their scope of practice to enable the student to meet their proficiencies and programme outcomes. Support and supervise students, providing feedback on their progress towards, and achievement of, proficiencies and skills AND have current knowledge and experience of the area in which they are providing support, supervision and feedback, and receive ongoing support to participate in the practice learning of students.

(NMC 2018c: 6)

Assessor roles

All students on an NMC approved programme are assigned to a different nominated academic assessor for each part of the education programme. Also all students on an NMC approved programme are assigned to a nominated practice assessor for a practice placement or a series of practice placements, in line with local and national policies.

(NMC 2018c: 8)

Academic assessors: responsibilities

Academic assessors collate and confirm student achievement of proficiencies and programme outcomes in the academic environment for each part of the programme and they make and record objective, evidence-based decisions on conduct, proficiency and achievement, and recommendations for progression, drawing on student records and other resources.

(NMC 2018c: 10)

One area you need to acknowledge is Duffy's research on the challenges in assessing students. Duffy identified a *'failure to fail'* poorly performing students by mentors/assessors (Duffy 2003; Duffy and Hardicre 2007). This has been exacerbated by the appeals process in universities, leading to mentors in the past not feeling able to fail students whose performance or conduct fell below an acceptable criterion because of the perceived bureaucracy of the system supporting students. While all students require support, even with appropriate supervision and fair assessment some students will still fail. It was concluded that responsibility for assessing students' competence resides not only with practice mentors but also with lecturers, course teams and management in both education and practice. This is an experience you have recently gone through. As you start to support your own students in practice it is worth remembering that while the students need support, your focus always must be protecting the public and maintaining the integrity of the profession.

However, sometimes mentors/supervisors do not give students thorough and regular feedback on their performance. Often this is due to concerns over the student's reaction and that it will be responded to with resistance and denial, or the assumption that this is subjective and biased. Wells and McLoughlin (2014) highlight that students cannot be aware of how to improve their performance unless they are given constructive, honest and timely feedback. In the past sometimes, mentors have assumed that poor performance will be addressed in future placements, leading to problems enduring, and students fell behind in their learning and professional development, or progressed when their competence ought to have been questioned sooner (Duffy and Hardicre 2007).

Therefore, the relationship between you as the student and your practice mentor/supervisor was crucial, not only to the success of your placement but the quality of learning. The student–mentor/supervisor relationship depends upon honesty, openness and trust. However, the student ought not be dependent and passive but seek to be assertive, commensurate to the student's level of competence and progress on the course. When you have students in your care you may come across this; reflect upon whether they are challenging you or challenging practice. If they are challenging you, ask why. It could be a learning experience for both of you.

The focus of FfP is around competency and the NMC's *Fitness to Practice* systems. There is also a focus on what constitutes unsafe practice and professional conduct which questions whether the educational component of pre-registration nurse training is sufficient (Killam et al. 2010). Much of the research attempts to clarify competency as opposed to understanding what constitutes incompetency under FfP. Several high profile cases have heightened the public's awareness of professionalism and safety, and the question of at what point the student is determined as being fit to practice. This is a vexed question, as pre-registration training seeks to prepare students to be fit for practice. While in contrast, the Trusts that host students and universities delivering the educational courses have procedures to determine whether a student is unfit for practice.

Reid (2010) suggests that the NMC continues to ask how certain students were ever allowed to complete and pass their nurse training. She suggests the clear documenting of all concerns, identifying problem students and managing them in a way that places equal value on both the academic and non-academic aspects of students being capable in areas of nursing practice such as leadership, which requires knowledge, attitudes and skill, and that where these are deficient students are considered a risk (King's College London 2009).

Activity 6.10

Looking back on your experiences of being a student:

What support that you were offered will you use with the students you support?

What support will you offer students that you did not receive?

How will you ensure failing students get the support they require?

What support will you ask for if you have to fail a student?

COMPETENCE IN CLINICAL PRACTICE

Following on from this, at qualification the Code (NMC 2018a) highlights the roles required.

> The Code contains the professional standards that registered nurses, mid-wives and nursing associates must uphold. Nurses, midwives and nursing associates must act in line with the Code, whether they are providing direct care to individuals, groups or communities or bringing their professional knowledge to bear on nursing and midwifery practice in other roles, such as leadership, education, or research. The values and principles set out in the Code can be applied in a range of different practice settings, but they are not negotiable or discretionary.

> (NMC 2018a: 3)

Using the NMC Code (2018a) nurses should:

- **Prioritise people**. You put the interests of people using or needing nursing or midwifery services first. You make their care and safety your main con-cern and make sure that their dignity is preserved, and their needs are recognised, assessed and responded to. You make sure that those receiving care are treated with respect, that their rights are upheld and that any dis-criminatory attitudes and behaviours towards those receiving care are challenged.
- **Practise effectively**. You assess need and deliver or advise on treatment, or give help (including preventative or rehabilitative care) without too much delay, to the best of your abilities, on the basis of best available evidence. You communicate effectively, keeping clear and accurate records and shar-ing skills, knowledge and experience where appropriate. You reflect and act on any feedback you receive to improve your practice.
- **Preserve safety**. You make sure that patient and public safety is not affected. You work within the limits of your competence, exercising your professional 'duty of candour' and raising concerns immediately whenever you come across situations that put patients or public safety at risk. You take necessary action to deal with any concerns where appropriate.
- **Promote professionalism and trust**. You uphold the reputation of your profession at all times. You should display a personal commitment to the standards of practice and behaviour set out in the Code. You should be a model of integrity and leadership for others to aspire to. This should lead to trust and confidence in the professions from patients, people receiving care, other health and care professionals and the public.

> (NMC 2018a: 6, 9, 13,18)

The nursing profession and the NMC wants you to be a nurse who is *Fit for Practice* by firstly successfully undertaking an NMC-approved registered nursing course, and at the end of your approved course being able to function as a full member of the NMC register and being fit for purpose, in managing both individual patient care and the ward environment. This means good conduct as well as good competence. You may be able to practise safely, but if you are unable to show integrity in your personal life, this could be a risk which may encroach on the professional arena. Examples have been highlighted on the NMC website (www.nmc.org.uk), and include inappropriate use of social media, civil and criminal convictions and discriminatory behaviour.

The Francis Report in February 2013, noted that between 2005 and 2008 conditions of appalling care were able to flourish in the main hospital serving the people of Stafford and the surrounding area (Francis 2013). The inquiry heard distressing personal stories, such as patients being left in their soiled bed clothes for lengthy periods and examples of improper feeding of patients (Francis 2013). Whilst the report makes for upsetting reading, the faults were not solely of the nursing staff at a clinical level, as a registered nurse had complained about the state of patient care within her department but had failed to follow the complaint through to a conclusion, and management had failed to investigate further.

What is apparent is that the Code (NMC 2018a), with its four main principles of prioritising people, practising effectively, preserving safety and promoting professionalism and trust, was not only weakly upheld, but in places missing altogether. The lack of professionalism and inadequate fitness to practise was extensive across the Trust. However, the report also suggests that there were a number of instances of managerial and director maladministration as some staff felt they were working in a culture of fear, mismanagement and secrecy which allowed poor practice to continue unquestioned. Interestingly, the Francis Report (2013) suggested in Recommendation 187 that

> Student nurses spend a minimum period of time, at least three months, working in the direct care of patients under the supervision of a registered nurse.
>
> (Francis 2013: 105)

This supervision should have occurred for you throughout your course. Kilcullen (2007) noted in her research that some students felt that they were inadequately supported in their clinical placements. You should have felt able to raise your concerns within the clinical area or with your personal tutor, if you thought you were not receiving the appropriate supervision for a third-year student.

Historically there have been a number of high profile cases across all fields of nursing which show lack of competence and conduct by individuals who are not fit to practice but also lack leadership skills in the clinical setting. The first case explored nationally was that of Beverley Allitt, who in 1991 gained employment soon after she qualified as an enrolled nurse on a children's' ward, even though she had a very significant sickness record. She went on to kill or harm a number of children with overdoses of medication or by suffocation until she was apprehended. It has been argued that she was not fit for practice even as a student due to her sickness record and her conduct while off duty and her training should have been discontinued. (See Clothier Report 1994 for further information.) This led to a number of changes in caring for children in the acute clinical area, which included two qualified nurses checking all medications, and more emphasis on the amount of sick leave students had taken during their nursing education.

Another nurse, Colin Norris, was convicted in 2008 of murdering four elderly female patients. At university he was considered to be an 'idle' student by his personal tutor during his three-year course and his tutor recalled having to warn him about his attitude and poor attendance (Stokes 2008). The university recorded Norris as having had 73.5 days absent (Beverley Allitt also had very poor attendance) but he was not considered unfit at the point of registration, even with the inquiry's findings that:

> Mr. Justice Griffiths Williams' 'Summing up to verdict' identifies that Colin Norris' attendance at clinical placements (caring for elderly people) was an ongoing problem and some placements refused to allow him to return. The result was that his training had to be extended. Witness statements also identify concern about his aggressive behaviour towards lecturers and the fact that on occasions he was found not to be telling the truth.

> (Proctor 2010: 4, 24)

The findings of the inquiries highlight a disconnection between the clinical and academic settings, with responsibility being placed upon the clinical area and practice supervisor. Indeed Proctor (2010) confirmed that placements were refusing to take Colin Norris. The question of responsibility for Norris fitness considering this attitude and manner illustrates the difficulties both mentors and personal tutors have when a student's professional behaviour is questioned. Sometimes it can be hard for mentors and lecturers to put into words their reservations or doubts about a student's attitude and suitability for entry onto the professional register.

Both Beverley Allitt and Colin Norris during their educational experience and once qualified were undermining professionalism and trust by abusing vulnerable patients who were thought by their families to be in a trusting environment, and therefore the patients and their families did not feel able to question their care. Both nurses did not maintain the reputation of the nursing profession, in their poor practice and behaviour both inside and outside work, and with the level of sick leave they had taken. However, a further issue is related to the lack of supervision and evaluation of their ongoing practice once qualified. As highlighted by Francis (2013), strong leadership is equally as important: if the ward had been monitoring the wellbeing of the patients, individually and as a group, the harm to patients may have been discovered more quickly (see **Chapters 8 and 9** on leadership and decision making where the issues are discussed in more detail).

Another example was the lack of professional integrity at Winterbourne View, which was a residential setting caring for twenty-four individuals who had learning disabilities, challenging behaviour or autism. While being staffed by a team of thirteen registered learning disability nurses, the care was largely 'led' by its biggest staff group of unqualified support workers. Training of all staff was 'skewed towards restraint practices with nothing about working with patients' (Community Care 2014: 1). As a result, the care needs of the clients were ignored, and any challenges from residents, family or friends were dealt with cruelly, or neglectfully.

The principles of the Code (NMC 2018a) were neglected: there was a failure to *prioritise people* – the patients' needs were ignored; there was a failure to *practise effectively* – restraint should always be the last resort; and there was a failure to *promote professionalism and trust* – the qualified staff let their leadership role lapse. The registered staff ignored the rights of the residents, maybe to avoid having challenging conversations about individual patients' human rights with the unqualified support workers. As students it may have been very difficult to go against the prevailing culture of the clinical area in which you were placed. However, once qualified there is a requirement to ensure not just your own but also your colleagues' behaviour demonstrates a professional and competent manner. Strengthening leadership should be a key focus of senior colleagues who have an obligation to spot and nurture talent, and this was reiterated in the Francis Report (2013):

> 1.188: Nurse leadership should be enhanced by ensuring that ward nurse managers work in a supervisory capacity and are not office bound. They should be more involved and aware of the plans and care for their patients [and students].
>
> (Francis 2013: 76)

The RCN pathway is a good approach to use as a guideline, and allows you to explore the risk for patients, yourself and others (RCN 2017, Figure 6.1). If you do not think that you are getting the support you require within the unit or clinical Trust, it is possible to seek further support, either from the NMC direct or from nursing unions. The health unions operate as independent agencies and exist to support and promote the needs, interests and wellbeing of students and qualified staff.

The NMC in their current documentation *Ensuring Public Safety, Enabling Professionalism* (2018d) highlight:

> we want fitness to practise to deliver improvements to the safe practice and professionalism of those who enter the process and not to curtail or restrict practice unnecessarily. We recognise that there will be situations where restrictions on or removal from practice are inevitable, but we don't think that these cases are the norm. Most registrants who have difficulties in their practice are willing and able to remediate the problem. We want to break down the barriers that stop them from doing so as early as possible.
>
> (NMC 2018d: 9)

Raising concerns step-by-step guide
Has the situation caused harm or distress or if you let the situation carry on, is it likely to result in harm or distress?

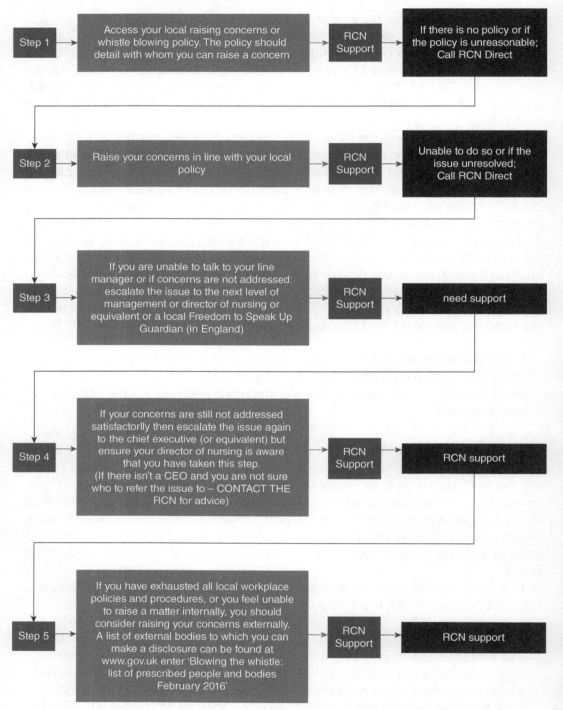

Figure 6.1   RCN (2017) Raising concerns step-by-step guide

Source: reproduced with kind permission of the Royal College of Nursing (2017) Raising Concerns, London: RCN

The NMC make it very clear, that all nurse have a responsibility to raise concerns, and escalate these concerns as quickly as possible:

Act quickly

If you think there is a risk that the nurse or midwife may pose to patients and the public, you should make us aware immediately. In some serious cases, it may be necessary for us to act quickly to stop the nurse or midwife from working or restrict their practice. Even if the risk is not immediate, please raise your concern as soon as possible with the nurse or midwife's employer if applicable. There is no time limit, but the longer ago an incident took place, the more difficult it is to investigate.

(NMC 2018d)

Ideally you should be able to work with your local management to follow up concerns about unsafe practice or inappropriate behaviour. If this is not possible you can contact the NMC confidentially either by phone, email or website. The NMC is unable to follow up concerns if they are not made aware of the issues. On the website all the forms are present and easy to access. Even if you are not sure, seek advice. It is far better to voice a concern than to worry about patient care. The NMC also makes the following points:

What we can't do

We can't make a nurse or midwife apologise to you or investigate general concerns about the nurse or midwife's place of work.

(NMC 2018d)

The NMC is not an intermediary service. Their role is to protect the public from misconduct or poor practice from nurses. It you require local support in a professional dispute then human resources may be the right service. If you have concerns about the whole organisation, then PALS or CQC may be the services to receive support. The NMC gives details of matters that it can investigate:

What we can consider

We can consider concerns that are serious enough to raise doubts about whether the nurse or midwife should be allowed to continue to practise as a registered professional, either with some form of restriction on their practice, or at all. Examples of allegations that we can investigate include:

- Abuse of professional position, for example an improper sexual relationship with a patient or service user, discrimination against patients and colleagues
- Serious or repeated mistakes in patient care
- Serious criminal offences
- Violence

- Dishonesty or fraud
- Serious breaches of patient confidentiality
- Serious concerns about a nurse or midwife's knowledge of the English language.

When we investigate, we consider:

- Whether the concerns are serious enough to raise concern about a nurse or midwife's fitness to practise
- Whether we can get evidence
- Whether the nurse or midwife has addressed the concerns.

(NMC 2018d)

It is always important to look at the context of the registered nurse's personal situation which has led up the incident. This must be professionally judged in the light of the seriousness of the allegations. The forms on the website and the guidance given provide clear instructions on how to report any of these incidents. Remember this is not just about what happens in the clinical area although this is the highest priority. Conduct when away from work is also relevant. Criminal activity of any type, including drink driving, theft and common assault should not be ignored. Also, civil issues such as dealing with social services due to concerns surrounding child care and neglect are also important. As nurses you should show kindness and compassion and support colleagues through this process whatever the outcome. The NMC also advises:

For self-referrals

If you're a nurse or midwife who needs to make a self-referral to us it's likely that we'll engage your employer when we investigate your referral. If you've not already discussed the issue you'd like to refer to us with your employer, then you should consider doing so.

(NMC 2018d)

It takes courage and insight to self-refer to the NMC: such behaviour could include one's incompetence, such as poor medicine management, conduct such as drink driving or health issues such as practising with poor eyesight. However, by referring yourself you are protecting the public and this awareness is clearly acknowledged by the NMC. The bravery shown alongside the insight will help to ensure that the most appropriate outcome for you and the safety of the public can be secured.

From the beginning of your course until you finish your nursing career you have a moral and professional responsibility to place patients and their families' requirements above any clinical or organisation issues. If you do not think that there is support for achieving the required outcomes for the patients then as a whistle blower, you should expect support from your superiors or managers. If this does not occur, then the NMC, or your nursing union, will be there to help.

All nurses have a role in supporting patients, and each other. As a qualified nurse you are the gatekeepers to future nursing students and your role will be to support, advise and assess students while safeguarding the needs of patients. This is a way to pass on the experiences you have had and to replicate the good role models of those who support you and help you learn from the challenges that you have experienced.

REFERENCES

Bray, L. and Nettleton, P. (2007). Assessor or mentor? Role confusion in professional education. *Nurse Education Today*, 27: 848–55.

Cassidy, S. (2009). Interpretation of competence in student assessment. *Nursing Standard*, 23: 39–46.

Clothier, C. (1994). The Allitt Inquiry: Independent Inquiry Relating to Deaths and Injuries on the Children's Ward at Grantham and Kesteven General Hospital During the Period February to April 1991.

CoDH/NMC Roundtable: The Future Focus of Nursing Education, March 2016. https://councilofdeans.org.uk/events/codhnmc-roundtable-the-future-focus-of-nursing-education/ accessed, August 2019.

Community Care (2014). Winterbourne View: A Case Study in Institutional Abuse. www.communitycare.co.uk.

Department of Health (1999). *Making a Difference*. London: Department of Health.

Duffy, K. (2003). Failing students: a qualitative study of factors that influence the decisions regarding assessment of students' competence in practice. Research report for the Nursing and Midwifery Council.

Duffy, K. and Hardicre, J. (2007). Supporting failing students in practice 1: assessment. *Nursing Times*, 103(47): 28–9.

Francis, R. (2013). Report of the Mid Staffordshire NHS Foundation Trust Public Inquiry. London: The Stationery Office.

Freshwater, D. and Stickley, T. (2004). The heart of the art: emotional intelligence in nurse education. *Nursing Inquiry*, 11: 91–8.

Gainsbury, S. (2010). Mentors passing students despite doubts over ability. NursingTimes.net [Online]. www.nursingtimes.net/whats-new-in-nursing/news-topics/health-workforce/mentors-passing-students-despite-doubts-over-ability/5013922.article, accessed 9 April 2014.

Goudreau, J., Pepin, J., Dubois, S., Boyer, L., Larue, C. and Legault, A. (2009). A second generation of the competency-based approach to nursing education. *International Journal of Nursing Education Scholarship*, 6: Article 15.

Holland, K., Roxburgh, M., Johnson, M., Topping, K., Watson, R., Lauder, W. and Porter, M. (2010). Fitness for practice in nursing and midwifery education in Scotland, United Kingdom. *Journal of Clinical Nursing*, 19: 461–9.

Hunt, L.A., McGee, P., Gutteridge, R. and Hughes, M., (2016) Manipulating mentors' assessment decisions: do underperforming student nurses use coercive strategies to influence mentors' practical assessment decisions? *Nurse Education in Practice*, 20: 154–16.

Huybrecht, S., Loeckx, W., Quaeyhegens, Y., Tobel, D.D. and Mistiaen, W. (2011). Mentoring in nursing education: perceived characteristics of mentors and the consequences of mentorship. *Nurse Education Today*, 31: 274–8.

Kilcullen, N.M. (2007). The impact of mentorship on clinical learning. *Nursing Forum*, 42: 95–104.

Killam, L.A., Montgomery, P., Luhanga, F.L., Adamic, P. and Carter, L.M. 2010. Views on Unsafe Nursing Students in Clinical Learning. *International Journal of Nursing Education Scholarship*, 7, 17.

King's College London (2009). Nursing competence: what are we assessing and how should it be measured? *Policy+ publication*.

MacLaren, J., Haycock-Stuart, E., McLachlan, A. and James, C. (2016). Understanding pre-registration nursing fitness to practise processes. *Nurse Education Today*, 36: 412–18.

National Nursing Research Unit (NNRU) (2009). Nursing competence: what are we assessing and how should it be measured? *Policy+ publication*.

Nursing and Midwifery Council (NMC) (2008). *Standards to Support Learning and Assessment in Practice*. London: NMC.

Nursing and Midwifery Council (NMC) (2009a). *Guidance on Professional Conduct: What Does the NMC Do?* London: NMC.

Nursing and Midwifery Council (NMC) (2009b). *Guidance on Professional Conduct for Nursing and Midwifery Students* [Online]. www.nmc-uk.org/Students/Guidance-for-students/, accessed 31 March 2014.

Nursing and Midwifery Council (NMC) (2014). *Standards for competence for registered nurses*. www.nmc.org.uk/globalassets/sitedocuments/standards/nmc-standards-for-competence-for-registered-nurses.pdf

Nursing and Midwifery Council (NMC) (2018a). *The Code: Professional Standards of Practice and Behaviour for Nurses, Midwives and Nursing Associates*. London: NMC.

Nursing and Midwifery Council (NMC) (2018b). *Future Nurse: Standards of Proficiency for Registered Nurses*. London: NMC.

Nursing and Midwifery Council (NMC) (2018c). *Realising Professionalism: Standards for Education and Training Part 2: Standards for Student Supervision and Assessment*. London: NMC.

Nursing and Midwifery Council (NMC) (2018d). *Ensuring Public Safety, Enabling Professionalism*. London: NMC. www.nmc.org.uk/globalassets/sitedocuments/consultations/2018/ftp/ensuringpublicsafety_v6.pdf

Ousey, K. and Gallagher, P. (2007). The theory–practice relationship in nursing: a debate. *Nurse Education in Practice*, 1: 199–205.

Proctor, S. (2010). Independent Inquiry into the Colin Norris Incidents at Leeds Teaching Hospitals NHS Trust in 2002. *Yorkshire and the Humber Strategic Health Authority*.

Reid, A. (2010). Identifying medical students at risk of subsequent misconduct. *British Medical Journal*, 340: 1041.

Royal College of Nursing (RCN) (2017). *Raising Concerns*. London: RCN.

Scott Tilley, D. (2008). Competency in nursing: a concept analysis. *Journal of Continuing Education in Nursing*, 39: 58–64.

Stokes, P. (2008). Colin Norris: from student to deadly abuser. *The Telegraph*, 2 March.

Stuart, C.C. (2007). *Assessment, Supervision and Support in Clinical Practice: A Guide for Nurses, Midwives and other Health Professionals*. Edinburgh and London: Churchill Livingstone/Elsevier.

Wells, L. and Mcloughlin, M. (2014). Fitness to practice and feedback to students: a literature review. *Nurse Education in Practice*, 14, 137–41.

Woodcock, J. (2009). Supporting students who may fail. *Emergency Nurse*, 16: 18–21.

7

Decision making and clinical governance

Mary Northrop

'The primary purpose of the NHS, and everyone working within it, is to provide a high quality service, free at the point of delivery to everyone who needs it. This common goal unites all those working in the NHS, from hospital doctors, to nurses, to GPs, to dentists, to allied health professionals, to clinical managers and non-clinical staff.'

(National Quality Board, 2011: 2)

This chapter will outline the importance of clinical decision making, in everyday care, and explore the tools and skills required for decision making concerning the care of individuals and groups of patients. Alongside clinical decision making an understanding of quality processes and the wider context in which this takes place is essential to provide evidence-based care. As newly qualified nurses, understanding how clinical decisions are made and developing the underpinning knowledge are part of the skill set for a successful career. This also includes developing an awareness of your own scope of practice and the need to work with the patient, their families and supporters, and the wider multi-disciplinary team. Underpinning this are the tenets of the 6Cs: Communication, Compassion, Care, Competence, Commitment and Courage (NHS England 2013).

Learning outcomes

- Understand the principles of decision making in clinical practice.
- Recognise your own boundaries and limits of competence.
- Demonstrate a problem solving approach to clinical decision making and application of appropriate concepts and tools.

- Reflect and evaluate your own application of decision making skills.
- Show awareness of the systems and processes related to clinical govern-ance and own contribution to ensuring the delivery of quality care.
- Understand the wider context of quality assurance and how this relates to person-centred care.

PRINCIPLES UNDERPINNING CLINICAL DECISION MAKING

Decision making is a key skill for both the care of individuals, but also groups of patients and ultimately for managing a clinical area. Successful decision making encompasses a wide range of skills and knowledge that will develop over time. Decision making is influenced by the context and circumstances within which it occurs, depending on:

- Presenting problem or condition of the patient
- Personal characteristics and experiences of the patient
- Environment in which care is taking place
- Resources and staffing
- Expertise and skills mix of the staff
- Policies and processes
- Cultural norms and values of the organisation
- Other factors unique to the situation.

Your ability to communicate underpins all stages of decision making. Effective communication with patients throughout their care will ensure relevant informa-tion is obtained and lead you to make appropriate plans and implement effective care. Communication is also important in developing a rapport with the patient and building trust and mutual understanding. Effective communication with the health care team encompasses good record keeping, handover of relevant infor-mation and collaboration.

Clinical decision making has direct effects on the patient, their support net-work and the health service in which they take place. The impact on the patient will be: physical, psychological, social and economic. For example, physically there is the potential for longer periods of ill health, complications including pain and discomfort, living on an ongoing basis with a debilitating health problem, the possibility of a decline in the capacity to perform everyday activities, and perhaps premature death. The psychological consequences include low mood or depression, increased stress and anxiety and loss of self-esteem or confi-dence. Social implications include pressures on relationships with other people including partners and family members, and, because of physical limitations, difficulties in continuing to participate in social relationships, friendships and work, resulting in social isolation. Financial problems may occur due to loss of income and difficulty in paying rent or mortgage and other bills. For the health service, the impact will be the increased cost of extended care delivery, potential insurance claims and the reputation of the service.

The Royal College of Nursing (RCN, 2008) produced a number of essential principles to consider when making decisions. These include:

- **Quality**: safety, dignity, effectiveness, efficiency and sustainability.
- **Accountability**: trust, transparency, leadership, confidentiality and responsibility.
- **Equality**: equity, diversity, accessibility, universality and advocacy.
- **Partnership**: consultation and negotiation, collaborative decision making, representation, legitimacy and involvement.

These principles underpin the organisational aspects of clinical decision making, with emphasis on clinical governance. Making clinical decisions for the care of individuals or groups in your care involves an understanding of laws, policies, guidance, processes and systems provided by the health care organisation to support the delivery and monitoring of care and ensuring that it is appropriate, and evidence-based.

CARE QUALITY COMMISSION AND LEGISLATION

The Care Quality Commission (CQC) was established in April 2009 with their role, and that of the organisations reporting to them, set down in the Care Quality Commission (Registration) Regulations (2009). The CQC is an independent regulator of health and social care in the United Kingdom (UK) whose jurisdiction includes the NHS, independent hospitals and care homes. Their role includes a variety of functions, ranging from registering care providers to monitoring, inspecting and rating services to safeguard patients and provide an independent voice on quality issues (CQC 2017a).

The CQC set out several fundamental standards that you and the health organisation providers you work for are required to meet. These include:

1. Person Centred Care: tailored to meet individual needs and preferences.
2. Dignity and Respect: individuals must receive care and treatment that upholds their dignity and ensures they are respected, including respecting privacy, equality and support to remain independent.
3. Consent: is required before undertaking care or treatment.
4. Safety: providers should not place individuals in situations that put them at risk of harm (that can be avoided) or give unsafe care or treatment. This includes ensuring that staff have the qualifications, competence, skills and experience to provide safe care and treatment.
5. Safeguarding from Abuse: individuals should not experience any type of abuse or improper treatment, including: neglect, degrading treatment, unnecessary or disproportionate restraint and inappropriate limits on freedom.

6. Food and Drink: individuals must be provided with enough to eat and drink to maintain good health while receiving care or treatment.
7. Premises and Equipment: the building and equipment used within it must be clean, suitable and maintained properly. The equipment must also be used properly.
8. Complaints: relevant systems need to be in place for individuals to make complaints. The complaints must be investigated thoroughly, and appropriate action taken.
9. Good Governance: appropriate systems and effective governance must be in place to ensure and check on quality and safety of care. This includes improving services and reducing risks related to health, safety and welfare.
10. Staffing: the provider must have enough suitably qualified staff to deliver care and treatment. They must be competent and experienced to undertake the care needed. Training and supervision must be given to help staff do their job.
11. Fit and Proper Staff: strong recruitment procedures are required, which carry out relevant checks to ensure appropriate individuals are employed who can provide care and treatment consistent with their scope of practice.
12. Duty of Candour: there ought to be an open and transparent attitude regarding care and treatment, including providing support and an apology if something goes wrong.
13. Display of Ratings: all providers must display their CQC rating where it can be seen, provide information on their website and make the latest CQC report available.

(CQC 2017b)

Activity 7.1

The fundamental standards and your own organisation

a. Look at one of the fundamental standards. How does your organisation address this?
b. Obtain a copy of your most recent CQC report. How easy was this to find? What were the main findings of the report?
c. Have any highlighted actions been addressed?

Alongside the monitoring of care delivery through the CQC you may have noted that some of the fundamental standards are underpinned by legislation. For example, the standards for premises and equipment are set out under the Health and Safety at Work Act 1974 (Health and Safety Executive, HSE) and more specific legislation, including the Lifting Operations and Lifting Equipment Regulations 1998 (LOLER) (HSE). Other standards, such as food and drink, and respect and dignity, are underpinned by guidance including the Essence of Care Benchmarks (DH 2010). For both areas of care, further guidance is available through the National Institute for Health and Care Excellence (NICE: www.nice.org.uk).

NICE guidelines relevant to own area of practice

NICE provides a range of evidence-based guidance for care delivery. Choose an aspect of care or treatment relevant to your own area for which there is a NICE guideline.

Reflect on how the guidance is implemented in your area of practice and if there are any aspects which could be incorporated into the current care provided.

Activity 7.2

CLINICAL GOVERNANCE

The CQC requires registered organisations and care providers to have robust governance systems to ensure that sufficient necessary resources are in place, the care and treatment provided is of a high quality and staff are adequately trained. Clinical Governance is the umbrella term for these systems and processes that work together to ensure high quality of patient care. Yet this all relies upon a pre-existent culture with a commitment to prioritising the delivery of excellent care. Clinical governance can be described as:

> ... the structures, processes and culture needed to ensure that healthcare organisations ... and all individuals within them ... can assure the quality of the care they provide and are continuously seeking to improve it.

(DH 2011)

Clinical governance in your own organisation

Find out the arrangements for clinical governance within your organisation.

Who are the post holders and what is their role?

What are the mechanisms for both raising issues and being informed of issues?

Activity 7.3

CLINICAL GOVERNANCE AND QUALITY

The focus on quality of care underpins clinical governance and how services are monitored and assessed. Defining quality in health care can be problematic as this can differ according to the patients' or professionals' viewpoint.

Mohammad Mosadeghrad (2013) suggests a definition which incorporates both viewpoints:

Consistently delighting the patient by providing efficacious, effective and efficient healthcare services according to the latest clinical guidelines and standards, which meet patient needs and satisfies [sic] providers.

(Mosadeghrad 2013: 215)

The World Health Organization (WHO) (2006) provides a working definition consisting of six dimensions (see Box 7.1).

Box 7.1   WHO, six dimensions of quality

Health care delivery needs to be:

- **Effective**, evidence based and producing improved health outcomes for individuals and communities
- **Efficient**, maximising resources and avoiding waste
- **Accessible** geographically and provided in a setting where skills and resources are appropriate to medical need
- **Acceptable and Patient-Centred**, taking into account the preferences and aspirations of individual patients and the cultures of their communities
- **Equitable** and taking into consideration personal characteristics such as gender, race, ethnicity, geographical location, or socioeconomic status
- **Safe** and minimising risks and harm to service users.

Source: WHO, 2006: 9

Activity 7.4

Ensuring quality

How do you think the quality of care might be measured? One example is the number of successful operations and the number of patients recuperating who achieve the hoped for level of functioning within the expected time.

Write down a range of different methods for measuring quality of care and then read the section below.

Within health organisations there are numerous methods for measuring and recording care. These include keeping statistics of reasons for care and treatment; the length of stay of patients on wards; and end point of treatment and patient satisfaction surveys. Quality of care can be measured in terms of the number of patients seen but also by the effectiveness of treatment and the success rate of recovery of patients. In some cases, patients will have illnesses from which they will not recover, and so the focus of treatment is instead on slowing the rate of deterioration. Therefore, the criteria used to measure care depend upon the intent and purpose for which the care is given. In some cases, the number of patients seen is not an indicator of success. A criticism often made of the NHS is that it is target led and focuses on high numbers and patient contacts as opposed to whether these contribute to the effective treatment of patients (Mooney 2010). As part of the measure of quality, the management of budgets and resources is also a requirement. Assessing whether services are meeting the needs of the population is ascertained by reviewing the statistical data relevant to the geographical area, which is then used to decide which services are needed and prioritised. The provision of services is also monitored through *Healthwatch UK*, which with input from local health watch groups, drawn from members of the public, evaluates services and is consulted on proposed changes. They have eight main principles, which the groups defined and gave concrete examples for (see Box 7.2).

Box 7.2 Healthwatch UK eight main principles 2018

Essential services

'I want the right to a set of essential prevention, treatment and care services, provided to a high standard which prevent me from being in crisis and lead to improvements in my health and care.'

Access

'I want the right to access services on an equal basis with others, without fear of prejudice or discrimination, when I need them and in a way that works for me and my family.'

Safe, dignified and high quality service

'I want the right to high quality, safe, confidential services that treat me with dignity, compassion and respect.'

Information and education

'I want the right to clear and accurate information that I can use to make decisions about health and care treatment. I want the right to education about how to take care of myself and about what I am entitled to in the health and social care system.'

(Continued)

(Continued)

Choice

'I want the right to choose from a range of high quality services, products and providers within health and social care.'

Being listened to

'I want the right to have my concerns and views listened to and acted upon. I want the right to be supported in taking action if I am not satisfied with the service I have received.'

Being involved

'I want to be an equal partner in determining my own health and wellbeing. I want the right to be involved in decisions that affect my life and those affecting services in my local community.'

A healthy environment

'I want the right to live in an environment that promotes positive health and wellbeing.'

Source: www.healthwatch.co.uk

For internal monitoring and evaluation of care, the most frequently used tools are clinical audit, which is discussed next.

CLINICAL AUDIT

Clinical audits enable the measurement of current performance, highlight good practice, which can be disseminated to all staff, and therefore improve practice and reduce errors. The audit cycle ensures that performance is measured against evidence-based benchmarks and, where performance gaps are identified, improvements can be implemented.

The audit cycle consists of the following stages:

- Preparing for audit
- Selecting criteria
- Measuring performance level
- Making improvements
- Sustaining improvements.

(Benjamin 2008)

Within your own organisation the preparation and selection of criteria that forms the basis of audit measures will be drawn from national standards (for example infection control standards are set by the Health and Social Care Act, 2008). Your involvement with the audit cycle as a nurse will start with measuring performance level. You will be required to undertake a variety of audits, with the most common being record keeping and hand washing following predetermined documentation and processes. The data collected is then fed back to the clinical governance team within the organisation to be collated, and then to establish if improvements are needed. Plans are then put in place to improve or maintain good practice. However, the onus is on individual practitioners to engage with this and enhance practice.

In the next section of the chapter risk assessment and management is discussed. This works alongside clinical audit and is an essential consideration in promoting patient safety and high standards of practice.

RISK ASSESSMENT

Within clinical areas there are a number of mandatory risk assessments. These include moving and handling but also environmental and certain specific clinical risks, while following an incident you may also have completed an incident form, commonly called a Datex sheet. In mental health settings it is routine practice to risk assess the propensity for self-harm or suicide for all service users. In all fields of nursing the assessment of deteriorating patients includes early warning systems where decisions are made based on physical observations and other factors.

As newly qualified nurses you will be developing management skills, which includes the need to be aware of a range of statutory and legislative guidance which impose certain requirements for how to respond in very specific situations. This includes Health and Safety legislation with regards to Controlled Drugs (Supervision of Management and Use) Regulations 2013 (DH), and RIDDOR (Reporting of Injuries, Diseases and Dangerous Occurrences Regulations) (2013), HSE (Health and Safety Executive 2013).

The content of the chapter, so far, has emphasised the issues and factors relating to the quality of care that is delivered. As newly qualified nurses it is essential to understand the organisational aspects, policies and processes, and legal and financial aspects that impinge on care. Ensuring that you are informed and equipped with the right information to deal with the various situations encountered in practice requires that you know where to find the information, and who to consult when unsure. The next part of the chapter draws on the information from the first part to focus on making clinical judgements and the skills and knowledge you are required to use.

MAKING CLINICAL JUDGEMENTS

Clinical judgement is informed opinion (using intuition, reflection and critical thinking) that relates observation and assessment of patients to identifying and evaluating alternative nursing options.

(Standing 2014: 7)

When you qualify as a nurse it is important that you are aware of the knowl-edge and skills needed to ensure competent clinical decision making and how these can be developed. These include competence in the delivery of patient care, taking in risk assessment, relevant and up-to-date clinical knowledge, communication skills, and delegation and leadership skills, rec-ognising own scope of practice, and being able to learn through experience. NHS Education for Scotland (n.d.) emphasise that good decision making will lead to safe care. They provide a continuum of decision making from simple to complex, with the former requiring intuition and experience, being high in volume and occurring daily. Complex decisions involve analytical skills, evidence-based practice, and the ability to synthesise previous experience. A combination of experience and skills will effectively facilitate the decision making process (see Box 7.3).

Box 7.3   NHS Education for Scotland: core skills of clinical decision making

- Pattern recognition: learning from experience.
- Critical thinking: removing emotion from your reasoning and being sceptical, with the ability to clarify goals, examine assumptions, be open-minded, recognise personal attitudes and bias, able to evaluate evidence.
- Communication skills: active listening – the ability to listen to the patient, what they say, what they do not say, their story, their experiences and their wishes, thus enabling a patient-centred approach that embraces self-management; information provision – the ability to provide information in a comprehensible way to allow patients or clients, their carers and family to be involved in the decision making process.
- Evidence-based approaches: using available evidence and best practice guidelines as part of the decision making process.
- Teamwork: using the gathered evidence to enlist help, support and advice from colleagues and the wider multi-disciplinary team. It is important to liaise with colleagues, listen and be respectful, whilst also being persistent when you need support so that you can plan as a team when necessary.
- Sharing your learning and getting feedback from colleagues on your decision making.
- Reflection: using feedback from others, and the outcomes of the decisions to reflect on the decisions that were taken to enhance practice delivery in the future. It is also important to reflect on your whole decision making strategies to ensure that you hone your decision making skills and learn from experience.

Source: NHS Education for Scotland n.d.: 3

The above principles will be addressed using the mnemonic ADDRESS:

- Assessment
- Decide
- Delegate
- Re-assess
- Evaluate
- Self-development
- Synthesis

ASSESSMENT

Assessment is the initial stage for most problem solving approaches including the nursing process. The Nursing and Midwifery Council (NMC) in the Code for Nurses and Midwives (2018) highlights that effective practice is underpinned by assessment which draws on evidence-based knowledge and best practice. This includes collaborating and communicating with the patient to ensure individualised care and with colleagues and members of the multi-disciplinary team (MDT).

What are the main assessment tools used within your own work setting?

Reflect on the assessment of a service user that you have undertaken.

What skills did you need to use?

Could you have improved how you carried out the assessment?

If yes how?

If no, why was the assessment successful?

Activity 7.5

Assessment needs to be holistic, considering psychological, physical, socio-cultural and economic factors regardless of the setting. When carrying out an assessment it is important that appropriate knowledge underpins the interpretation of diagnostic tools and observations that are collated. Understanding of the parameters of observations in relation to the service user (including age, ethnic or religious factors), pathophysiology, pharmacology and current guidance will permit the interpretation and influence the actions that are taken.

The importance of assessing both physical and mental health in all areas of nursing cannot be ignored. Physical assessment includes base line observations but also the activities of daily living, which include: breathing, communicating, maintaining safety, eating and drinking, elimination, maintaining body tempera- ture, sleep and rest, personal cleansing and dressing, work and leisure, sexuality, and death and dying (Peate 2010). Whereas mental health assessment includes: appearance and behaviour, speech, mood, thoughts, perception and insight. In addition, assessments of anxiety, sleep and nutrition are needed (Fallon, P. and G. 2017) to ascertain how the mental state may be impacting on the physical state. Assessment also relies on input from others and it is essential to ascertain the patient's views and those of relatives and carers. Insights from others as to how an individual's behaviour and mood differs from normal can add to the base line but also help to build a fuller picture.

Comprehensive and detailed assessment is part of the nursing process. Without a holistic approach, clinical decisions may not include relevant fac- tors or the subtle and nuanced way in which some needs are evident, and therefore the actions that are taken may not be appropriate. How this relates to the NMC code is discussed in more detail in **Chapter 6** on fitness to prac- tice. Figure 7.1 identifies a range of factors to consider when making clinical decisions.

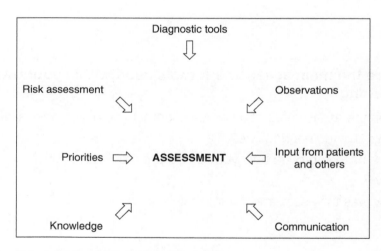

Figure 7.1   Decision making: assessment

The type and number of diagnostic tools used will differ depending on your field of nursing, clinical setting, speciality and the degree of urgency. Early Warning Scores are common across nursing settings to identify the deteriorating patient and there are tools for nutritional assessment. In adult and child settings the ABCDE tool (Resuscitation Council 2017; Edwards and Coyne 2013) may be used (Airway, Breathing, Circulation, Disability and Exposure). The assessment of children will also consider the developmental stage, and its impact and influ- ence on health (Edwards and Coyne 2013).

Diagnostic tools

List the different diagnostic tools used in your area of practice and what they assess.

Which work the most effectively, why?

Which is the least effective, why?

DECIDE

Once a full assessment has been made the next stage is to decide what needs to happen. In some instances, assessment may have included the use of an Integrated Care Pathway which will automatically recommend the actions to take. In emergency situations the decision will be to provide care to prevent further deterioration and safeguard the individual. This may also mean that as a newly qualified nurse your first decision is that the situation is not within your current ability and needs to be escalated. The SBAR communication tool has been proven to enable essential information to be handed over:

- **S-ituation** – a concise statement of the problem
- **B-ackground** – pertinent and brief information related to the situation
- **A-ssessment** – analysis and considerations of options; what you found or think
- **R-ecommendation** – action requested or recommended; what action you want

(Institute for Healthcare Improvement 2017)

For non-emergency situations decisions need to be made for care to be delivered in a timely fashion. Figure 7.2 includes some of the considerations when deciding on what course of action to take.

Sometimes what we may regard as a care priority may not be the same for the patient. For example, a patient may feel that looking after their pet is of greater importance than the treatment they need. The decisions that are made concerning care need to involve the patient's perception and knowledge of the condition. Providing clear and jargon-free information and explanations about the treatment options will help this process, as will listening and demonstrating empathy and respect. Person-centred care also involves informed consent as a fundamental principle and includes the communication of the risks and benefits of treatment.

Alongside service user preferences, decisions about care ought to also consider the availability of resources and what options are available. Once decisions are agreed the next stage is to ensure these are documented in the care plan (planning stage of the nursing process) and to meet record keeping guidelines

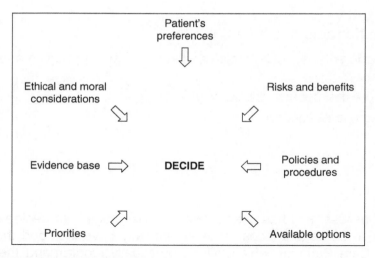

Figure 7.2   Decision making: decide

as set by the NMC's Code for Nurses and Midwives (NMC, 2018). The next stage is to put the plan into action (implementation stage), which includes the delegation of tasks to appropriately skilled and knowledgeable staff.

DELEGATE

During your management placements as a student nurse you would have started to develop delegation skills through managing a group of service users. As you progress in your career this skill will be developed to include managing a clinical area or case load. There are many factors that need to be considered when delegating, and it is important to be able to communicate effectively with those you are asking to undertake the task. Figure 7.3 provides a summary of the factors and skills required. Delegation requires understanding of the care environment, the roles and abilities of those you work with and whether delegation is appropriate.

When delegating it is important to ensure that the member of staff to whom you are delegating has the knowledge and skills required to undertake the task, and the capacity within their current workload. The Royal College of Nursing (RCN) provides a useful guide to delegation (RCN 2011). They stress that delegation includes a duty of care and is only appropriate if it is in the best interest of the service user. Whether the person carrying out the delegated action is a registered nurse or health care assistant, as the registered nurse you are accountable for the care given and should only undertake the task if you have the relevant skills, knowledge and expertise. The development of good communication skills for delegating to others is an essential skill as a newly qualified nurse. An assertive approach combined with an explanation as to why the individual has been

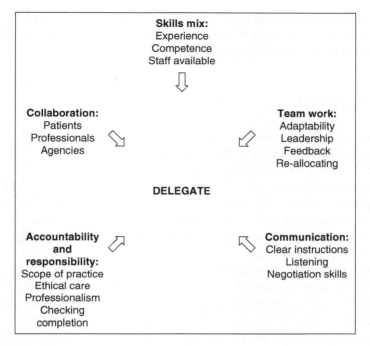

Figure 7.3   Decision making: delegate

selected to carry out the task is essential. It is then important to listen if they have any concerns or questions, and to ensure that they have understood what is required. Part of delegation is also to state the time requirement and how the completion of the task needs to be fed back.

Allocation of staff

In your own area of practice, what are the factors that you need to consider when allocating the care of a group of service users?

Activity 7.7

Your answer may include:

- The patient's condition, and level of care required.
- Person-centred care considering patient preferences and routines.
- The skills mix of the staff and their experience.
- How many staff need to be allocated to meet the needs of the patients and to ensure their safety and that of staff members.
- Other demands that may impact on the care, for example tests, ward rounds, and admissions and discharges (inpatient care) or travel distances (community care).

Once care has been decided on and implemented the next stage is to consider the impact, and if the options have been successful. This moves into the evaluation stage of the nursing process.

RE-ASSESSMENT

To evaluate care there is a need to re-assess both the situation and the progress in relation to the care plan or integrated care pathway. Re-assessment can be ongoing, particularly in fast-moving scenarios. For example, if a deteriorating patient is given oxygen the effects can be assessed within a short time frame. In mental health, crisis intervention can prevent an individual self-harming. Observations, either physical or psychological, enable a picture to be formed as to how interventions are or are not working. These may be carried out continuously, or at brief set intervals.

As with assessment, re-assessment needs to be patient-centred, to ensure that the care you give is meeting assessed needs, and explained to the patient so that care is collaborative and carried out transparently and with an awareness of accountability. Based on the re-assessment the care may be changed or adapted. It is essential that informed consent is respected, and that the nurse accepts the service user's wishes to refuse care or treatment.

The other aspect of re-assessment relates to the management of care and feeds back into delegation, teamwork and resources. Communication with the team delivering the care contributes to understanding what is happening and how the service user is responding, while collating information from all parties, both verbal and written, will aid in making future decisions (see Box 7.4).

Box 7.4   Good practice: handover and delegation

George was in charge of the morning shift. The staff on duty received the handover from the night shift which highlighted the main issues and which service users were higher priority. Based on the information, George allocated qualified staff to monitor those seen as at higher risk. All staff were asked to assess their allocated service users, while ensuring that breakfast and other tasks were carried out.

Following breakfast, George spoke to all the staff and then re-allocated based on the assessment. This may have included patients whose condition was deteriorating and needed a more experienced nurse, or new admissions who required further investigations such as EEGs, which required someone not only skilled to undertake the investigation but able to work alongside the doctor looking at the treatment required following the results.

The above shows the importance of re-assessment to ensure the right person, with the right knowledge and skills, is caring for the right service user. It also highlights that an individual's health needs can change, and care provision needs to be adapted.

EVALUATE

The evaluation of care can be ongoing, as well as at the end of a shift or when an individual's care is completed. Evaluation of an individual's care may include a patient satisfaction survey which will focus on the wider services provided and informal evaluation through feedback from the service user. It also involves looking at what worked and what did not work and why (evaluation stage of the nursing process). This incorporates the clinical decisions made, evidenced through nursing records.

For emergency situations, **Critical Incident Analysis** is a useful tool as it enables those involved to consider what went well and what could have been changed. When this is done well it also acts as a support learning process for those involved. Ghaye and Lillyman (2010) provide a list of experiences that may potentially be critical incidents:

- An incident that is an ordinary experience.
- An incident where the experience did not go to plan (positive or negative experiences).
- An incident that went well.
- An incident that reflects the values and beliefs held by the individual.
- An incident that identifies the contribution of qualified practitioners.
- An incident that allows the identification of learning.

A further learning opportunity is using case study presentations to examine the care given and underpinning evidence-based practice.

Evaluation of management skills includes reflecting on your own practice and feedback from others. Schön (1996) describes three types of reflection:

- Knowing-in-action
- Reflecting-in-action
- Reflection-in-practice

The first, *knowing-in-action*, relates to knowledge that you apply at that time, for example, your knowledge of how to delegate. The second aspect, *reflecting-in-action*, relates to the ability to think while doing and adapting your own actions to meet the current situation. For example, you may be dressing a wound and realise that you need to change the type of dressing. A second example is that you may be communicating with a service user and you note that they do not appear to understand what you are saying and realise that your approach needs to be altered and you need to change the language being used. *Reflection-in-practice* is looking at your practice and examining different aspects. Schön (1996) suggests that because much of practice is repetitive or similar you can become burnt out and see what you expect to see, rather than what is there. By reflecting-in-practice you may be able to recognise where the use of tacit knowledge may be affecting practice and correct this. Schön also suggests reflection-in-practice includes both looking at the situation when it is occurring (reflection in action) and looking back at practice (reflection on action).

Feedback from others can be both formal and informal. Some organisations use a 360° evaluation approach which involves getting feedback from managers, peers and others. All this feeds into self-development.

SELF-DEVELOPMENT

In your role as a registered nurse you will be constantly learning and developing new skills to enhance your practice. In the evaluation section, reflection was outlined and its use illustrated in relation to specific events and to examining your own practice. Reflection can be informal or use a more formal but appropriate model. The importance of reflection has been embedded in the re-validation process as operated by the NMC (2017) and is linked to appraisal.

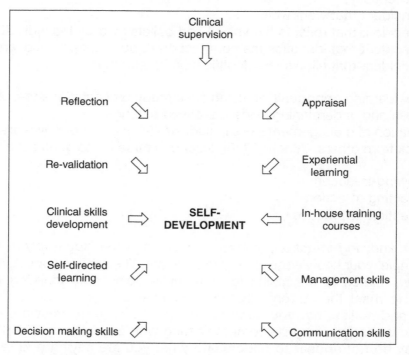

Figure 7.4   Decision making: self-development

Figure 7.4 suggests a range of forms of self-development which can be tailored to your requirements and that of your speciality and the organisation. Formal learning includes keeping up to date with mandatory training and applying for courses which develop specialist knowledge to enhance practice. As student nurses you will have been exposed to a range of clinical skills. Your first experiences as a qualified nurse will enable you to further develop these in relation to the needs of the specialities and patient groups. The NMC Code (2015) stresses the importance of maintaining knowledge and skills but also ensuring that care is evidence-based.

Part of self-development is the ability to analyse (Bloom's Taxonomy of Learning level 4: Gershon 2015). Analysis involves understanding a range of information and drawing conclusions about what is effective and what is not. A useful tool to establish what you need to develop is a Strength/Weakness/Opportunities/Threats (SWOT) analysis (Pearce 2007). This involves identifying strengths, weaknesses (areas that need to be developed), opportunities available (formal or informal learning and within the organisation) and threats that may affect the ability to learn or develop (organisational change, role change and workload). Having completed a SWOT analysis this can be shared during supervision and at appraisal to inform a personal development plan.

Self-development SWOT

Think of a learning need that you have.
Now work through the stages of SWOT one at a time.
Write down your notes in your professional portfolio

Activity 7.8

SYNTHESIS

Synthesis is the level 5 stage of Bloom's taxonomy (Gershon 2015) and brings your knowledge, skills and experience together creatively to be able to apply what was learnt to different situations. This can be likened to *'thinking outside the box'*, or finding innovative approaches to care from disparate types of information.

Carper (1978 cited in Risjord 2010) identified what she considered to be nursing knowledge ('ways of knowing') under four categories:

- **Empirics**: research-based knowledge
- **Ethics**: moral and ethical knowledge
- **Aesthetics**: how to provide care
- **Personal knowledge**: own experiences and intuition.

Nurses bring these aspects together to inform decision making when providing care. Active learning that focuses on empirics will develop why you do what you do, but needs to be combined with the other 'ways of knowing' to ensure care is carried out in a caring and compassionate way.

Activity 7.9

Synthesis: Carper's 'ways of knowing'

Reflect on the care you provided for an individual.

How did you incorporate the four categories of knowledge?

Reflect on the management of a group of patients.

How did you incorporate the four categories of knowledge?

Compare the two reflections, what were the differences and similarities?

Another important way in which decision making skills can be developed is through observing others. Social learning theory (Bandura 1977 cited by Sternszus and Cruess 2016) states that role modelling has four stages:

- **Observation** of the role model
- **Developing** a mental representation of what was observed
- **Reproducing** the behaviour
- **Incorporating** the behaviour into your own work.

Activity 7.10

Social learning theory

Think of an individual who has influenced your practice, and who you will try to emulate.

What is it about them that you want to emulate?

Use the SWOT criteria to identify how you might develop your learning in this respect.

What practical steps can you take to add some of these skills to your capabilities?

Knowledge and skills need to be shared through nurturing and teaching others. During preceptorship you are guided by a knowledgeable and experienced professional. However, this is also a reciprocal arrangement where you bring your own knowledge and skills which may inform their practice. You will act as a role model for other members of the team and be supporting student nurses with a view to becoming mentors or supervisors in the future. Part of leading a team is to identify the strengths of all the members, and any gaps that could impact on the quality of care. Encouraging team members to develop skills and supporting them in the process is an important part of the role of the qualified nurse as a leader.

This chapter has provided an overview of clinical decision making and a range of factors that influence the requisite skills. The chapter started by considering the context of care and the importance of organisational systems and quality processes under the umbrella of clinical governance. The role of external bodies (CQC and Healthwatch UK) in acting as useful advocates and monitors of health care provision was also acknowledged. Within the chapter it was established that it is essential that newly qualified nurses become well acquainted with the legal and regulatory frameworks and standards that operate in their specialist areas of practice to deliver high standards of care.

The second part of the chapter focused on the development of clinical decision making and the requisite knowledge and skills. The use of the mnemonic ADDRESS links to the principles of decision making, the use of a problem solving approach and the tools that can be utilised. It is important to reiterate that you need to be aware of your own knowledge and skills and when you need to seek help or escalate situations to others. This applies throughout your career not just the transition from student to registered nurse. At the heart of your practice is the service user and the responsibility to provide safe, informed, quality care.

REFERENCES

Benjamin, A. (2008). The competent novice audit: how to do it in practice. *British Medical Journal*, 36: 1241–5.

Care Quality Commission (CQC) (2017a). *Who We Are*. www.cqc.org.uk/about-us/our-purpose-role/who-we-are, accessed 4 October 2017.

Care Quality Commission (CQC) (2017b). *Fundamental Standards*. www.cqc.org.uk/what-we-do/how-we-do-our-job/fundamental-standards, accessed 4 October 2017.

Department of Health (DH) (2010). *Essence of Care 2010: Benchmarks for the Fundamental Aspects of Care*. www.gov.uk/government/uploads/system/uploads/attachment_data/file/216691/dh_119978.pdf, accessed 4 October 2017.

Department of Health (DH) (2011). *Clinical Governance Guidance*. www.gov.uk/government/news/clinical-governance-guidance, accessed 4 October 2017.

Department of Health (DH) (2013). *Controlled Drugs (Supervision of management and use) Regulations 2013 Information about the Regulations*. www.gov.uk/government/uploads/system/uploads/attachment_data/file/214915/15-02-2013-controlled-drugs-regulation-information.pdf, accessed 5 October 2017.

Edwards, S. and Coyne, I. (2013). *A Survival Guide to Children's Nursing*. E-book. Edinburgh: Churchill Livingstone. www.dawsonera.com/readonline/9780702047077, accessed 4 October 2017.

Fallon, P. and G. (2017). The nature and types of assessment. In M. Chambers (ed.), *Psychiatric and Mental Health Nursing: The Craft of Caring*, 3rd ed. Abingdon: Routledge, pp. 143–51.

Gershon, M. (2015). *How to Use Bloom's Taxonomy in the Classroom: The Complete Guide*. N.p.: Learning Sciences International.

Ghaye, T. and Lillyman, S. (2010). *Reflection: Principles and Practices for Healthcare Professionals*, 2nd ed. London: Quay Books

Health and Safety Executive (n.d.: a). *The Health and Safety Act 1974*. www.hse.gov.uk/legislation/hswa.htm, accessed 4 October 2017.

Health and Safety Executive (n.d.: b). *Lifting Operations and Lifting Equipment Regulations 1998 (LOLER)*. www.hse.gov.uk/work-equipment-machinery/loler.htm, accessed 4 October 2017.

Health and Safety Executive (2013). *RIDDOR – Reporting of Injuries, Diseases and Dangerous Occurrences Regulations 2013*. www.hse.gov.uk/riddor/, accessed 5 October 2017.

Institute for Healthcare Improvement (2017). *SBAR Tool Kit*. www.ihi.org/resources/Pages/Tools/sbartoolkit.aspx, accessed 5 October 2017.

Mooney, H. (2010). Poor training, staff cuts, and overemphasis on targets led to failures at Stafford, says inquiry. *British Medical Journal*, 340(7745): 501.

Mosadeghrad, M. A. (2013). Healthcare service quality: towards a broad definition. *International Journal of Health Care Quality Assurance*, 26(3): 203–19.

National Quality Board (2011). *Quality Governance in the NHS: A Guide for Provider Boards*. www.gov.uk/government/uploads/system/uploads/attachment_data/file/216321/dh_125239.pdf, accessed 4 January 2017.

NHS Education for Scotland and Effective Practitioner (n.d.). *Clinical Decision Making*. www.effectivepractitioner.nes.scot.nhs.uk/media/254840/clinical%20decision%20making.pdf accessed 16 July 2017.

NHS England (2013). *Compassion in Practice: One Year On*. www.england.nhs.uk/wp-content/uploads/2016/05/cip-one-year-on.pdf, accessed 30 September 2017.

Nursing and Midwifery Council (NMC) (2015). *The Code for Nurses and Midwives: Professional Standards of Practice and Behaviour for Nurses and Midwives*. London: NMC. www.nmc.org.uk/standards/code/read-the-code-online/#third, accessed 2 March 2017.

Nursing and Midwifery Council (NMC) (2017). *Welcome to Re-validation*. http://revalidation.nmc.org.uk/welcome-to-revalidation/, accessed 28 October 2017.

Nursing and Midwifery Council (NMC) (2018). *The Code, Professional Standards of Practice and Behaviour for Nurses, Midwives and Nursing Associates*. www.nmc.org.uk/concerns-nurses-midwives/fitness-to-practise-a-new-approach/

Pearce, C. (2007). Ten steps to carrying out a SWOT analysis. *Nursing Management*, 14(2): 25.

Peate, I. (2010). *Nursing Care and the Activities of Living*, 2nd ed. Chichester: Wiley-Blackwell.

Resuscitation Council (2017). *The ABCDE Approach*. www.resus.org.uk/resuscitation-guidelines/abcde-approach/, accessed 5 October 2017.

Risjord, M. (2010). *Nursing Knowledge: Science, Practice, and Philosophy*. Chichester: Wiley-Blackwell.

Royal College of Nursing (RCN) (2008). *Principles to Inform Decision Making: What Do I Need To Know?*, 2nd ed. https://my.rcn.org.uk/__data/assets/pdf_file/0009/78696/003034.pdf, accessed 16 July 2017.

Royal College of Nursing (RCN) (2011). *Accountability and Delegation: What You Need To Know*. https://my.rcn.org.uk/__data/assets/pdf_file/0003/381720/003942.pdf, accessed 5 October 2017.

Royal College of Nursing (RCN) (2015). *Accountability and Delegation: A Guide for the Nursing Team*. https://my.rcn.org.uk/__data/assets/pdf_file/0006/627216/004852_HP-A-and-D_pocketguide_June2015.pdf, accessed 16 July 2017.

Schön, D. (1996). *The Reflective Practitioner: How Professionals Think in Action*. Aldershot, Ashgate.

Standing, M. (2014). *Clinical Judgment and Decision Making for Nursing Students*, 2nd ed. London: Sage.

Sternszus, R. and Cruess, S. (2016). Learning from role modelling: making the implicit explicit. *The Lancet*, 387(10025): 1257–8.

World Health Organization (2006). *Quality of Care: A Process for Making Strategic Choices in Health Systems*. www.who.int/management/quality/assurance/QualityCare_B.Def.pdf, accessed 4 October 2017.

PART III

Next phases

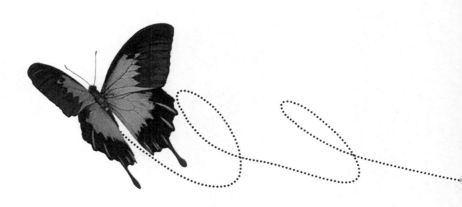

PART II

Next phases

8

Continuous professional development (CPD) and revalidation

Chris Thurston

Part of your commitment to the NMC (2018) code is to:

'19.2 take account of current evidence, knowledge and developments in reducing mistakes and the effect of them and the impact of human factors and system failures.'

Caring for patients and clients and their families is a demanding and important role, and this chapter will help you as a qualified nurse to develop the skills and expertise to practise compassionately and effectively. The chapter will help you to learn how to provide specialist care while at the same time transforming existing nursing qualifications by using a personal development plan (PDP).

Learning outcomes

- Defining and planning for CPD for the first year and beyond.
- Personal development and lifelong learning.
- Career development and planning.
- Revalidation.

When you had your interview, you would have asked what career opportunities were available in the clinical setting, and what you could potentially achieve in learning experiences. Now you have settled into your clinical environment in your chosen area, it may seem time to relax, knowing you have completed a significant event in your professional journey. This is a little naive as you may have soon realised that you are learning just as much if not more than you did as a student nurse. You and your preceptor may have discussed the first steps during induction and the mandatory study days required. You will also have discovered the need to learn the advanced communication skills required to support the patient as part of the multi-professional team; you may be the person in charge on occasion, or the leader of a team of professionals. As your experiences progress, undertaking audits and managing staff and resources may also be part of your role. The other area of knowledge which is as important is the area of practice itself. You may be in an acute clinical area, working in the community or an outreach service such as in a prison or hospice.

Firstly, you need to practise self-compassion to maintain your ability to provide compassionate care. You are already aware of the relationship between caring for yourself and caring for others to support patients and their families effectively. Secondly, and just as importantly is the requirement to continue to develop knowledge and expertise in your chosen area. Every clinical area whether in the hospital, a tertiary setting, community or exceptional or unusual setting has unique interventions. This may be because of the types of clients or patients, such as a child in a hospice, or an environment with patients who may have also offended as in a forensic mental health unit. Other areas may be rarer such as caring for passengers on a cruise ship or clients attending a private aesthetic clinic. Therefore, your own development portfolio and continuing personal development (CPD) will be unique. If you can develop and maintain good record keeping for your clinical work and learning experience, this will aid you in your revalidation, which we will explore more closely later in the chapter.

Activity 8.1

What regular routines do you undertake to support your mental and physical wellbeing?

Examples could be exercise, swimming or the gym or walking.

How often are you able to share at work or home the challenges you have faced during your working day?

Find out what resources in your clinical area or Trust are available for you in terms of supervision, support groups or social activities.

CONTINUING PROFESSIONAL DEVELOPMENT (CPD)

This is how you maintain and improve your leadership skills, while broadening your clinical and theoretical knowledge, and also enhance your personal and professional qualities. Using a systematic approach encourages ongoing professional competence and conduct. This needs to be linked to your lifelong learning, while acknowledging that your everyday practice has the realistic potential for new learning experiences and using your reflections to enhance patient care.

CPD is defined by the Health and Care Professional Council (HCPC) as follows:

> CPD provides the opportunity for you to raise meaningful questions in relation to your specialism; and to discover an awareness to develop solutions and the ability to communicate these processes.

(HCPC Registration)

The HCPC go on to give some very simple examples of events that you may experience in practice which may help to give evidence of lifelong learning and professional development (see Table 8.1).

Table 8.1   Events in practice to give evidence of lifelong learning and professional development

Work-based learning	Professional activities	Formal/ educational	Self-directed learning
Learning by doing and written reflection of the event	Involvement in a professional body or specialist-interest group	Courses related to your current practice area	Reading journals or articles
Filling in self-assessment questionnaires	Lecturing to or teaching junior colleagues	Further education maybe in a broader field such as management	Reviewing books or articles
Reflective practice including case studies, and writing these up as a record	Mentoring/ supervising/ assessing students and junior colleagues	Research issues and area of interest in your practice area	Updating your knowledge through the internet or TV
Audit of service users and act on the results	Being an examiner/ tutor link to your local Trust or university	Attending conferences on areas of practice or research aligned to your practice	Keeping a portfolio of your progress
Coaching from others	Undertaking revalidation	Writing articles or papers	
Discussions with colleagues, both nursing and multi-professional	Organising journal clubs or other specialist groups	Going to seminars	

(Continued)

Table 8.1   (Continued)

Work-based learning	Professional activities	Formal/ educational	Self-directed learning
Peer review another practice or specialist knowledge	Maintaining or developing specialist skills (for example, musical skills)	Distance or online learning	
Gaining and learning from clinical experience and reflecting on these	Being an expert witness	Going on courses accredited by a professional body	
Involvement in the profession-related work of your employer (being a representative on a committee)	Giving presentations	Planning or running a course	
Work shadowing colleagues whose role is of interest to you	Organising accredited courses		
Secondments to other areas of clinical, research, or academic practice	Supervising research or students		
Job rotation with your own unit, or across the Trust	Being a national assessor		
Significant analysis of events you have experienced	Project work		
In-service training	Expanding your role such as liaising with other groups such as service users or advocate groups		

Source: adapted from HCPC, 2019

Activity 8.2

Reflecting on Table 8.1, list the activities you already undertake.

Also using Table 8.1, decide which activities you would like to develop further.

Your area of practice will dictate to some extent the CPD you may wish to undertake. All clinical areas will have mandatory study dates and annual trainings which will help to keep you up to date and should be included in your portfolio. If, for example, you are working in critical or acute care you may be recommended to undertake a post-registration and/or postgraduate course in critical or acute care. In the example of critical care there is a requirement from the clinical area to have a significant number of qualified staff with specific specialist qualifications to ensure sufficient numbers of staff have up-to-date knowledge and expertise in the clinical work area (a minimum of 50 per cent of registered nursing staff will be in possession of a post-registration award in Critical Care Nursing). This may mean that the unit will support you both financially and with study leave. This is becoming less common as Trusts have less resources for education and training as funding is diverted to direct patient care.

An example for nurses in adult acute care may be a course which explores aspects of acute and critical care and the support required for family or carers. The teaching would be guided by the Department of Health (2009) competencies for the acutely ill adult. National reports such as *Time to Intervene* (HQIP 2012) and *Time to Act* (Parliamentary Ombudsmen 2013) continue to record failings in the provision of acute health care provision. Therefore, as a nurse you may have to acknowledge that individuals have the right to specialist care, regardless of location or speciality. Patient safety is an absolute priority, including maintaining adequate tissue perfusion and oxygenation essential for life. Courses and study days will help you if this is your field of nursing to understand both the concepts required and the physiology behind the process. If you are a practitioner in this area you need the knowledge necessary to care for the highly dependent and acutely ill patient.

In previous chapters safeguarding has also been discussed; specialised knowledge of this may be a requirement in some areas of practice including children's nursing and mental health and learning disabilities. Other specialised areas of knowledge related to practice include applying the Mental Health Act 2007 using evidence-based practice. The latest review highlighted the challenges faced by health professionals supporting people with mental illness or mental health issues (Department of Health 2018).

It is important for your professional development for you to prioritise which courses and study days are significant to you. They may also be a priority to your unit or Trust; this would be ideal as they would be more likely to support your request to undertake the studies. However, it is important to think of your own professional journey, and some of your choices, such as a course which is not directly related to your current practice, may be more important for you. Therefore, you may need to look at the pros and cons for these priorities. You may want to undertake a higher degree, but are unable to receive funding from your employer. Do not give up on this, rather explore other resources such as charities and nursing funds which can offer part or complete funding. Some examples are given below.

The Queen's Nursing Institute

This is a registered charity dedicated to improving the nursing care of people in their own homes and communities. See www.qni.org.uk/help-for-nurses/educational-grants/.

Research Council funding

The seven UK Research Councils represent one of the most important sources of postgraduate funding in the UK. It is their job to provide support for research projects and for the training of potential new researchers. Though most of their resources are now directed towards PhD programmes, you can sometimes receive Research Council funding for Master's degrees – particularly 1+3 or New Route PhD programmes. These begin with a taught Master's degree in the first year, followed by a three-year PhD programme. Funding usually covers course fees and a tax-free maintenance grant. See www.findaphd.com/funding/guides/research-council-studentships.aspx.

Erasmus funding

The European Commission's Erasmus+ Programme is not specific to the UK, but it *does* support students to study abroad at universities across Europe (and beyond). You can study at multiple universities with a Joint Master's Programme scholarship. See www.findamasters.com/funding/guides/erasmus-joint-masters.aspx.

Charities and alternative funding sources

You may be surprised to learn that a lot of funding for postgraduate study is actually available from charitable trusts and learned societies. All sorts of organisations are interested in helping to promote new research and training in particular fields and for talented postgraduates. Grants from charities and similar organisations tend to be relatively small – between £100 and £1,000 on average – but there's no reason why you can't combine lots of them to cover your costs. In fact, this approach to financing postgraduate study has become so popular it even has its own name: 'portfolio funding'. See www.findamasters.com/funding/guides/charities.aspx.

University scholarships

It is important not to overlook the assistance that might be offered by the institution where you are going to study your higher degree. Universities are keen to encourage and support good applicants to their postgraduate programmes and some will have significant financial resources available to help them do this. Investigating university scholarships for postgraduate funding usually means getting in touch with institutions and asking what kinds of support they offer.

You can also apply for RCN bursaries, RCN Foundation bursaries and Mary Seacole awards to fund your professional development:

RCN bursaries: can help fund courses, study tours, projects, research and conference attendance.

Mary Seacole awards: the awards fund projects that aim to improve the health outcomes of black and minority ethnic communities.

More funding options: Explore more funding options that could support your continuing professional development. See www.rcn.org.uk/professional-development/scholarships-and-bursaries.

Education for Health

One of the benefits of studying with Education for Health are the guides to funding opportunities. These are available from a variety of sources: charities, external organisations, pharmaceutical companies and employers. Take advantage of their industry links and advice to help to secure potentially valuable funding for training. As a charity, they work hard to keep costs to a minimum and this is reflected in the prices for their courses. Sometimes they also offer Education for Health bursaries, and always update details of these on their website when available. See www.educationforhealth.org/education/courses/funding-sponsorship/.

Funding streams: charity scholarships

This PDF highlights different organisations which can offer funding and support: www.jpaget.nhs.uk/media/220097/funding-streams-registered-nurses-and-midwives.pdf.

Postgraduate studentships

Consult the experts on the specialist postgraduate platform, a range of services connecting intending postgraduate students and universities with study and funding opportunities on offer. See www.postgraduatestudentships.co.uk.

PERSONAL DEVELOPMENT PLAN USING A PORTFOLIO

One way to keep order in your collection of written evidence is by using a personal portfolio. A portfolio is simply a way to house records showing you have completed studies including your revalidation requirements. This is needed for you to keep your evidence systematically together. For all nurses this should include practice hours, reflections, peer reviews, and evaluation by others including patients, colleagues and students. This is a good starting point when you are preparing for revalidation. However, this should be a continuous developmental process of your career progression rather than a task to undertake three years after you qualify. The way you store the information is up to you. Traditionally this was achieved by paper in folders; now there are online resource to logically keep things together. See both the RCN and the NMC websites:

RCN link: www.rcn.org.uk/professional-development/your-career/nurse.

NMC professional development: www.rcn.org.uk/professional-development/your-career/nurse and http://revalidation.nmc.org.uk/news.html.

Both the RCN and the NMC give clear advice about how to compile the evidence. All nurses are required to undertake continuing professional development activities to maintain, update and improve their knowledge and practice, and they can use their portfolio to document these activities. Creating and maintaining a portfolio can also enable nurses to identify their strengths and learning needs, and to develop a learning plan to address these needs. A portfolio can assist nurses to store and manage their revalidation or re-registration documents in one place, so that these can be easily updated and produced when required, for example in performance reviews and job applications.

The portfolio is, however, so much more than providing evidence for your revalidation. The ability to reflect on your practice and to be able to apply new knowledge you have gained through informal or formal learning is greater than the revalidation process alone. The revalidation process is important to enable the NMC to be confident in the competence and conduct of the current nurses on the register, and to be able to offer assurance to the general public and interested parties that nurses are undertaking up-to-date and evidence-based practice. You should see this as the minimum standard you may achieve. However, to excel in your care for patients and their families you need to strive for more learning experiences.

Welp et al. (2018), in their research highlighted the importance of reflecting on practice by asking 244 nurses via questionnaires to examine the relationships between participation in personal professional development activities and the mediating and moderating effects of reflective thinking and perceived usefulness of development activities. The results seem very sensible in that the more current your professional development is, the more likely you are to work better in teams and to have higher performance levels. This is not just about having more skills or knowledge, although that is important, it is also about the enhanced skill to reflect on your practice.

> Personal professional development activities enhance reflection in and on practice as these activities were linked with higher perceived quality of care and teamworking. It is important to ensure that the positive effects of personal professional development activities should target nurses' professional development needs and need to be perceived as useful by those who undertake them.
>
> (Welp et al. 2018: 3988)

What is clear from the research is that the study or personal development you undertake must be seen to be useful to you, not just the area of clinical practice you are working within (see Figure 8.1).

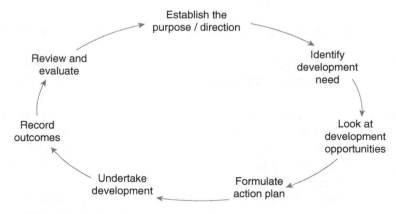

Figure 8.1   Personal development cycle

Source: CMI Personal Development Cycle (2019) Copyright © 2019 Chartered Management Institute (CMI) www.managers.org.uk

ACTION CHECKLIST

Establish your purpose or direction

The purpose of any development activity needs to be identified.
  This involves:

- Gaining an awareness of your current standing and future potential within your chosen clinical setting.
- Exploring what you are good at, interested in and what motivates you.
- Taking account of the organisational realities you may encounter.
- Linking your plans to organisational needs as much as possible.
- Recognising the characteristics of the kind of clinical work that fits with your value system.

(Adapted from CMI Personal Development Cycle, 2019)

Use the guidance and headings above to establish your personal purpose and direction.

Activity 8.3

Identify development needs

The identification of development and learning needs for you in practice may emerge from intended or actual new clinical tasks or management responsibilities, or from dissatisfaction with current clinical routines.

- Some people know what they are good at in practice, others may be less sure.
- Various instruments such as self-assessment tests, benchmarking exercises and personal diagnostics are available to help you assess your skills in a structured way.
- Your development needs will depend largely upon your career goals: will you stay in this clinical area or will you spread out to other areas?
- If you intend to remain in a similar clinical area, you may need development to re-motivate or re-orient yourself, or improve your current performance and effectiveness.
- Alternatively, development may be required to prepare you for promotion, your next job or a career move.

(Adapted from CMI Personal Development Cycle, 2019)

Activity 8.4

Use the guidance and headings above to identify you own development needs.

Identify learning opportunities

As a result of one, or several, of the assessment processes above, draw up a list of the skills or knowledge you need to acquire, update or improve. Compare this list with your current skills and knowledge base and identify the gaps.

Activity 8.5

Use the guidance above and Table 8.2 to identify your own learning needs and opportunities.

Table 8.2   Examples for identifying your own learning needs and opportunities

Skills or knowledge you need to acquire, update or improve	Current skills and knowledge base	Identify the gaps
E.g. Specialist safeguarding knowledge	*General safeguarding knowledge*	*Specific knowledge in regard to clinical area of practice*

Your learning styles are important as you may learn best by trying out new things or prefer to sit back and observe; you may prefer to experiment or carry out research.

Follow this web link to a questionnaire to help you identify your own learning styles: Research Notes, P. Honey and A. Mumford, *The Learning Styles Questionnaire*, ELN resources: http://resources.eln.io/honey-mumford-learner-types-1986-questionnaire-online/ (accessed January 2019).

Activity 8.6

YOUR DEVELOPMENT

In addition to your own Trust or clinical area, consider government and private advisory agencies, literature and open learning, multi-media or online packages, professional institutes, your peer groups, networks and colleagues, and family and friends.

The range of learning options available can be broadly differentiated into three categories:

- Education takes place over a sustained but finite period of time, usually leads to a qualification and may open the way into a new career direction.
- Training is carried out at a specific time and place and is usually vocationally relevant and limited to specific measurable aims and objectives.
- Development encompasses a wide range of activities with learning potential that are either work-based (such as work shadowing, job rotation, secondment, attachment, mentoring, delegation, counselling or coaching) or personal (such as private reading, authorship, presenting papers, peer group contacts, networking, or community involvement).

There will be occasions when unplanned development opportunities arise, such as a last minute vacancy on a course or a place at an event, which will require you to take account of your priorities when considering whether to follow up on that opportunity.

(Adapted from CMI Personal Development Cycle, 2019)

Formulate an action plan

For each of the skills and knowledge gaps you identify, set yourself development objectives. These need to be

- SMART: Specific, Measurable, Achievable, Realistic and Timely. There must be an element of challenge in them so that they stretch you as an individual and carry you on to new ground.
- Attainable and viable within a realistic time-frame, otherwise time will overtake you.

Activity 8.7

Using Table 8.3 as an example, undertake your own SWOT analysis of your strengths and needs for further learning in your clinical area.

Table 8.3 Examples of SWOT Analysis

Strengths	Weakness
E.g. Good verbal and written communication skills	E.g. Not sure how to use spreadsheets and other IT software
Opportunities	**Threats**
E.g. In-house computer courses and online modules	E.g. Not being freed from regular duties to attend the study sessions

Activity 8.8

Using the SMART targets below as an example, undertake your own assessment for learning to develop your own SMART action plan.

Specific, Measurable, Achievable, Realistic and Timely

Undertake the development

Put your plan into action.

- What you do and how you do it should be your choice.

In addition to training courses, options include:

- Work shadowing: you could explore both nursing and other professional colleagues.

- Secondment: this may be within the Trust or further afield if you could arrange reciprocation.
- Job rotation: this is especially helpful if you are new to an area or have patients from another area in the Trust.
- Project work: this is a good way to explore a specific area of practice over a longer period of time and will both benefit your knowledge but also enhance patient care.
- Networking: make use of every opportunity to discuss with others in your field of interest.
- Community involvement: health is a broader interest than health professional concerns: become involved in patient groups or community programmes

(Adapted from CMI Personal Development Cycle, 2019)

> While undertaking more formalised courses is important, think with the help of the list above of any other activities you could undertake to further your learning, career development or insight into your clinical area.

Activity 8.9

Record the outcomes

Keeping records of all activities serves to remind you and others, such as potential employers, what you have done. Most importantly, your records will help you to focus on what you have got out of your development activity. Elements to be recorded include:

- The date
- The development need identified
- The chosen method of development
- The date(s) when development was undertaken
- The outcomes
- Further action needed

(Adapted from CMI Personal Development Cycle, 2019)

Evaluate and review

Evaluation is the key stage in the self-development cycle. There are two issues you should reflect upon.

- Whether the development activity you have undertaken was appropriate and worthwhile.
- Whether and how your skills or working behaviour have improved as a result.

Evaluating development activities also involves asking the following questions:

- Did I give feedback to the educator/lead?
- Did I gain constructive criticism from the educator/lead?
- What am I able to do better in practice as a result of undertaking the activity?
- Has this experience thrown up further clinical development needs?
- How well did this development method work for my specific learning style?
- Could I have gained more from this activity?
- Would I follow this approach again and if not how would I do it differently?

(Adapted from CMI Personal Development Cycle, 2019)

Activity 8.10

It is important to know whether learning opportunities you have taken have achieved the outcome you wanted or expected.

Reflect back on the most recent education you have received; did it live up to your expectations?

If it was better than you expected why was that? An example may be that it has enhanced your practice more than you thought it would.

If it was less successful, for example not relevant to practice or poorly taught, how would you ensure better learning experiences in the future?

Evaluation will also provide a key lead for the next stage of the continuing cycle. Goals change, tasks may vary, and new learning needs will emerge. It is important to revisit and revise your own plan at regular intervals.

(Heading and content for this section adapted from CMI, Copyright © 2020 Chartered Management Institute, www.managers.org.uk/knowledge-bank/personal-development-planning)

REVALIDATION

Revalidation is the process that allows us to maintain our registration with the NMC. It builds on existing arrangements for the renewal of that registration. As part of this process, you need to meet a range of requirements designed to show that you are keeping up to date and actively maintaining your ability to practise safely and effectively. You need to collect evidence and maintain records to demonstrate to a confirmer that you have met the revalidation requirements (http://revalidation.nmc.org.uk/index.html)

Every three years you will be asked to apply for revalidation using the NMC online system as a means of renewing registration. Completing the revalidation process is our own responsibility as nurses and midwives. You are the owners of your own revalidation process. Revalidation is not an assessment of your fitness to practise, or a new way to raise fitness to practise concerns or an assessment against the requirements of your current or former employment. The purpose of revalidation is to improve public protection by making sure that you demonstrate your continued ability to practise safely and effectively throughout your career (http://revalidation. nmc.org.uk/index.html).

One of the main strengths of revalidation is that it encourages you to use the Code (NMC 2018) in your day-to-day practice and personal development. Revalidation includes requirements that encourage you to seek feedback from patients, service users and colleagues. It requires you to consider the role of the Code in practice by having a reflective discussion with another nurse or midwife and seeking confirmation that you have met those requirements from an appropriate person. It will encourage you to engage in professional networks and discussions and reduce professional isolation (http://revalidation.nmc.org. uk/index.html).

THE REQUIREMENTS

450 practice hours

The hours that count towards this requirement are those in which you rely on your skills, knowledge and experience as a registered nurse or midwife. This may include providing direct care to patients but can also include managing teams, teaching others and helping to shape or run a care service. I used my teaching and managing of nurse tutors for my 450 hours.

- You are required to undertake 450 hours of nursing practice over a three-year period.
- Your practice hours reflect your current scope of practice, but they do not have to be related to your original field of practice when you first joined the register.
- The NMC have a template to help you record your practice hours.
- The NMC provides some examples that you might find helpful.
- There is also guidance for you what to do, including with respect to dual registration

(Adapted from http://revalidation.nmc.org.uk/index.html)

35 hours of CPD including 20 hours of participatory learning

You must have undertaken 35 hours of CPD relevant to your scope of practice as a nurse or midwife in the three-year period since your registration was last renewed, or when you joined the register. Of those 35 hours of CPD, at least 20 must have included participatory learning. I used both my mandatory study sessions at the university and the sessions I attended for my own personal development and nursing research interests; I had homework from some of this learning along with personal reflections I undertook.

You must maintain accurate records of CPD you have undertaken. These records must contain:

- The CPD method.
- A description of the topic and how it related to your practice.
- The dates on which the activity was undertaken.
- The number of hours (including the number of participatory hours).
- The identification of the part of the Code most relevant to the activity.
- Evidence that you undertook the CPD activity, including certification if relevant.
- To meet the participatory learning requirement, you simply have to undertake activity that involves interaction with one or more other professionals.
- This can be in a physical environment or a virtual one.
- Examples of participatory learning can include:
  - Attending a conference
  - Taking part in a workshop
  - Attending a relevant training course
  - Undertaking a course or module.
- Remember to keep evidence of your CPD to show to your confirmer.
- Use the NMC template to help you record your CPD.

(Adapted from http://revalidation.nmc.org.uk/index.html)

Five pieces of practice-related feedback

You must have obtained five pieces of practice-related feedback in the three-year period since your registration was last renewed or you joined the register. I used feedback from my manager, students and peers who gave me a 360 degree feedback about my performance over the previous three years. As a nurse or midwife, it is likely that you already receive a range of feedback, and the five pieces of feedback you collect can come from a variety of sources and in a variety of forms.

- It can be written or verbal, formal or informal.
- It may come from patients and service users, colleagues and management.
- It can also include feedback from team performance reports or your annual appraisal.

We recommend that you keep a note of the content of any feedback you receive, including how you used it to improve your practice. You can use the NMC template to help you record your feedback. Be careful not to record any information which may identify another person.

(Adapted from http://revalidation.nmc.org.uk/index.html)

Five written reflective accounts

You must have prepared five written reflective accounts in the three-year period since your registration was last renewed or you joined the register. As a nurse tutor and manager, I have found it useful throughout my career to keep a reflective journal. This enables me to draw out from this the five reflective accounts required.

Each reflective account must be recorded on the approved form and must refer to:

- An instance of your CPD, and/or
- A piece of practice-related feedback you have received, and/or
- An event or experience in your own professional practice
- And how they relate to the Code.

The NMC wants to encourage you to reflect on your practice, so you can identify any improvements or changes to your practice as a result of what you have learnt. Each of your five reflections can be about an instance of CPD, feedback or an event or experience from your work as a nurse or midwife – you can even write a reflection about a combination of these. It is important to think about the Code when you write your reflections and consider the role of the Code in your practice and professional development.

- The NMC has provided a form which sets out the different things you need to think about when writing your reflections. You **must** use this form to record your written reflective accounts.
- The NMC has provided some examples of completed reflective accounts that you might find helpful in thinking about how to approach the requirement. These accounts don't need to be lengthy or academic-style pieces of writing.
- You should be careful not to record any information in your reflective accounts which may identify another person.

(Adapted from http://revalidation.nmc.org.uk/index.html)

Reflective discussion

You must have had a reflective discussion with another NMC registrant, covering the five written reflective accounts on your CPD and/or practice-related feedback and/or an event or experience in your practice and how this relates to the Code. I discussed my validation process with a colleague; this was someone I trusted to be supportive but also objective during the process. You must ensure that the NMC registrant with whom you had your reflective discussion signs the approved form, recording their name, NMC PIN, email, professional address and postcode, as well as the date you had the discussion

- The reflective discussion can be one of the most rewarding elements of revalidation.

- This discussion could be with someone who works with you on a regular basis, but you can decide who they will be.
- The NMC has produced a guidance sheet which contains some useful information to help you to get the most out of this discussion.
- The discussion should take place face to face and you should be careful not to discuss other individuals in a way that can identify them.
- If your confirmer is a nurse or midwife, your reflective discussion can form part of the confirmation discussion.
- If your confirmer is not a registered nurse or midwife, you must have your reflective discussion before your confirmation discussion takes place.
- The NMC has provided a form which you **must** use to record your reflective discussion.

Although you are not required to submit this form to the NMC at any point, you should keep it safe as part of your records. You may choose to store the completed reflective discussion form in either paper or electronic format. Please make sure you respect the fact that this form contains personal data about your reflective discussion partner.

(Adapted from http://revalidation.nmc.org.uk/index.html)

Health and character declaration

This requirement asks you to declare that your health and character are sufficiently good to enable you to practise safely and effectively, and to declare any cautions or convictions.

- You must provide a health and character declaration.
- You will be asked to declare if you have been subject to any adverse determination that your fitness to practise is impaired by any other professional or regulatory body.
- You must declare if you have been convicted of any criminal offence or issued with a formal caution.
- You don't need to collect evidence to prove you meet this requirement; you just need to complete the declarations when making your application.
- If you are declaring a caution or conviction, see the NMC main website

(Adapted from http://revalidation.nmc.org.uk/index.html)

Professional indemnity arrangement

As a registered nurse or midwife, you are legally required to have a professional indemnity arrangement in place in order to practise. Most employers provide the appropriate cover for their employees, but it is worth checking with your employer to confirm this. For my declaration within the university this was supported by the faculty.

- You must declare that you have, or will have when practising, appropriate cover under an indemnity arrangement.

- If you are self-employed you will need to have arranged your own professional indemnity cover.
- You don't need to provide evidence to prove you meet this requirement.
- You need to confirm you have the appropriate cover when making your application.
- For more information on professional indemnity, read the NMC guidance document.

(Adapted from http://revalidation.nmc.org.uk/index.html)

Confirmation

This will be a declaration in which you have demonstrated to an appropriate confirmer that you have complied with the revalidation requirements. The NMC has provided a form for you to use to obtain this confirmation. The NMC has also produced specific information for confirmers and you should share this with your confirmer before you meet, so that they understand what they are being asked to do.

- The NMC will ask you for information for the purpose of verifying the declarations you have made in your application.
- The NMC will ask you to provide the name, NMC PIN or other professional identification number (where relevant), email, professional address and postcode of the confirmer.
- The role of a confirmer is an important one.
- This is the person who looks at the evidence you have collected and 'confirms' that you have met the revalidation requirements.
- When the time comes, it's important that you try to speak to your confirmer face to face, as you'll need to talk them through how you have met all of the requirements.
- You should obtain your confirmation in the final year of your three-year renewal period, to ensure that it is as recent as possible.
- Where possible, your confirmer should be your line manager.
- Your confirmer does not need to be a registered nurse or midwife and does not need to be the same person you had your reflective discussion with, although this can often be a sensible choice as it makes the process a little easier.
- The NMC has provided a form which you **must** use to record your confirmation. Although you are not required to submit this form to the NMC at any point, you should keep it safe as part of your records. You may choose to store the completed confirmation form in either paper or electronic format.
- Please make sure you respect the fact that this form contains personal data about your confirmer, and that you uphold your obligations in relation to confidentiality and data protection.
- The NMC has examples to identify an appropriate confirmer.
- If you do not have a line manager, or access to an NMC-registered nurse or midwife, you can seek confirmation from another health care professional who is regulated in the UK. For example:

- Art therapist
- Biomedical scientist
- Chiropodist
- Chiropractor
- Clinical scientist
- Dentist
- Doctor
- Dietician
- Hearing aid dispenser
- Occupational therapist
- Operating department practitioner
- Optician
- Optometrist
- Orthodontist
- Orthoptist
- Osteopath
- Paramedic
- Pharmacist
- Physiotherapist
- Psychologist
- Podiatrist
- Prosthetist / orthotist
- Radiographer
- Social worker
- Speech and language therapist

If you are not sure if your confirmer can sign your declaration, contact the NMC directly and seek advice.

(Adapted from http://revalidation.nmc.org.uk/index.html)

This chapter will be useful for both starting you on your professional journey and reminding you to keep up to date both for supporting your current practice with patients and their families and to keep a record of your professional reflection and learning for revalidation. This will be an ongoing process which will encourage you to be a lifelong learner and an advocate both for your patients and yourself. You will not be able to offer a high standard of care if you are not supported by a high standard of management, both clinically and in senior management. Always place the needs of the patient first, and do not forget your own needs for support, compassion and guidance.

I always keep my portfolio up to date and this has enabled me to quickly access information for applying for jobs, courses or qualifications. The process of revalidation was very straightforward and the person who undertook the reflections was a colleague who knew the work I had undertaken over the last three years. The process of maintaining up-to-date practice regardless of the area of practice you are working in is important for you, but more importantly for the patients, clients or indeed students you work with.

REFERENCES

Chartered Management Institute (CMI). *Personal Development Planning*. www.managers. org.uk/knowledge-bank/personal-development-planning, accessed January 2019.

Department of Health (2007). *Mental Health Act 2007*. London: HMSO.

Department of Health (2009). Framework of Competencies for Recognising and Responding to Acutely Ill Patients in Hospital: Consultation Report. London: HMSO.

Department of Health (2018). *Independent Review of the Mental Health Act*. London: HMSO.

Faculty of Intensive Care Medicine and Intensive Care Society (2013). *Core Standards for Intensive Care Units*.

Health and Care Professional Council (HCPC) (2019). www.hcpc-uk.org/registration accessed 22 October 2018.

Healthcare Quality Improvement Partnership (HQIP) (2012). *Time to Intervene*. National Confidential Enquiry into Patient Outcome & Death.

Honey, P. and Mumford, A. ELN resources. http://resources.eln.io/honey-mumford-learner-types-1986-questionnaire-online/, accessed January 2019.

Nursing and Midwifery Council (NMC) (n.d.). *Revalidation*. http://revalidation.nmc.org. uk/index.html accessed January 2019

Nursing and Midwifery Council (NMC) (2018). *The Code:* Professional Standards of Practice and Behaviour for Nurses, Midwives and Nursing Associates. www.nmc.org. uk/standards/code/.

Parliamentary Ombudsmen (2013). *Time to Act*. London: HMSO.

Welp, A., Johnson, A., Nguyen, H. and Perry, L. (2018). The importance of reflecting on practice: how personal professional development activities affect perceived teamwork and performance. *Journal of Clinical Nursing*, 27(21–22): 3988–99.

9

Leadership and management

Chris Thurston and Nick Wrycraft

Pepin et al. (2010) define clinical leadership as:

> '...a professional competency demonstrated in clinical care that galvanizes the nurse to influence others to continuously improve the care they provide.'
>
> (Pepin et al. 2010: 269)

In organising the delivery of nursing on inpatient wards it is common for one qualified and experienced staff nurse to be the nurse in charge for a period of duty, and to lead a group of staff, including peers on the same grade. Often this role is rotated from one shift to another among several staff nurses on a unit. Being in charge permits nurses to exercise their skills leading a team and provides the opportunity to maximise their effectiveness in delivering good quality care to patients. Further emphasis upon leadership as a crucial function of nurses and health care professionals has been provided by the recommendations of recent reports regarding failings in the organisation of health care (Francis Report, 2013; Keogh Review, 2013). Therefore, developing an effective understanding of leadership and becoming competent and capable to lead a shift and be the nurse in charge is essential learning in making the transition from student to newly qualified nurse.

This chapter explores how leadership and management are essential functions of the role of the newly qualified nurse in practice. Developing leadership and management skills will improve not only the personal effectiveness of the nurse but the teams within which they work.

Learning outcomes

- The concept of leadership and clinical leadership in nursing.
- Theories and styles of leadership.
- The management skills required to effectively organise the care of a group of patients.

THE CONTEXT OF LEADERSHIP IN THE NHS

In recent years there have been several high profile reviews and reports into catastrophic failings in care. These include the Francis Report (2013), about failings in patient care in Mid Staffordshire NHS Foundation Trust; the Keogh Review (2013), which led research on fourteen failing trusts with high mortality rates; and the Berwick Report (2013), which came up with specific recommendations on improving patient care and how to support patients, families and staff to enhance the care process. All the reports recommended reforming and modernising the delivery of health care and crucially enhancing clinical leadership of staff at all levels. In addition to this the NHS Constitution (2015) represents a clear commitment to the rights and expectations of patients as recipients of health services and the expectations of staff reinforcing the notion of health care services as accountable to the public.

As the most populous profession within health care (Willis Commission 2012), and through being at the centre of the delivery of multi-disciplinary care, nurses are well situated to promote leadership within the health care workforce. Intensifying the focus on the preparation and training in leadership of pre-registration nurses therefore has great potential to promote high standards and positively influence the effectiveness of delivery of patient care.

The recommendations of the Willis Commission (2012) outline a number of interesting initiatives about nurses of the future. These include widening the range of entry points for staff to become qualified nurses, ensuring that graduate nurses are trained to lead teams, and an emphasis on applying critical thinking skills to practice. These ideas reflect an intention to integrate leadership as a central competence in the practice of nurses. While qualified nurses have traditionally combined a leadership role in organising and coordinating the work of peers, and simultaneously managing junior colleagues, in the future there will be an increased emphasis on performing this role through working with colleagues in a greater variety of roles

LEADERSHIP

Effective leaders act with others to pursue and achieve a shared goal (Whitehead et al. 2010). Within this understanding the leader exerts their influence upon others to initiate and bring about change, or attain a specific goal (Sullivan and Garland 2010; Northhouse 2018). Therefore, leaders are catalysts who marshal and concentrate resources, including people and materials, to produce an intended and desired outcome.

Common perceptions of leadership perceive it to be apparent in bold actions, heroism and significant actions, with the leader performing a prominent role in events. In some situations, clear and assertive leadership is needed. Yet often in nursing, leadership is a more circumspect and subtle skill. Leaders promote team-working, and value the skills and contribution of team members. This activity is apparent in conversations, interpersonal interaction, and how, and on what activities, time and resources are allocated. Therefore, leadership is a subtle and nuanced skill which is flexible and adaptable.

Activity 9.1

Think of an example you have seen in practice of good leadership.
Now consider, what was good about it?
What did the leader do?

Theories of leadership examine features of the leader and various aspects of the relationship between the leader and situations in which they are involved. Some theories focus on the disposition and attributes of the leader (for example trait theory), while others emphasise the situation in which the leader is active (such as contingency theory), or the nature of the goal or change to which they are committed. Both perspectives can be correct, as there are attributes or personal characteristics which many leaders have and can be generally agreed as being effective in leading people; for example, being able to use adaptable skills in communication to tailor messages and instructions in accordance with the different needs of individuals. Skills such as being able to monitor multiple situations at the same time which are specific to leading a nursing shift often take time to develop and cultivate through repeated exposure and experience. Yet in other cases, for example a crisis or emergency, the nature of the situation necessitates that the leader has certain specific skills or attributes.

TRAIT THEORY

Trait theory suggests that individuals possess specific characteristics or attributes which exert an impact on leadership. Traits rely on human characteristics and responses.

When is permission needed to undertake activities?

When you oversee a team caring for a group of patients, what activities can be undertaken by individuals in the team without discussion and what activities need to be either discussed or permission sought for.

Looking at Table 9.1, which traits do you possess?

Table 9.1 Examples of trait characteristics

Trait in relation to clinical practice	High level of the trait	Low level of the trait
1. Openness	• Creative approaches to clinical practice • Open to trying new experimental treatments • Focused on tackling new challenges • Happy to think about abstract concepts	• Dislike change of clinical routine • Do not enjoy new approaches to care or management • Not very imaginative when exploring different options with patients • Dislike abstract or theoretical concepts
2. Conscientiousness	• Spend time preparing for all patient interventions • Finish important tasks right away and able to prioritise • Pay attention to details • Enjoy having a set schedule for the patient's care and treatment	• Dislike structure and schedules and argue each situation has a tailor-made solution • Make messes and not take care of things • Procrastinate important tasks and unable to prioritise • Fail to complete the things as they are supposed to be done
3. Extraversion	• Enjoy being the centre of attention and happy to lead a team • Enjoy meeting new people including patients and families • Feel energised when they are around other people • Say things before they think about them	• Dislike being the centre of attention and may have difficulty leading a team • Prefer solitude • Find it difficult to start conversations especially challenging conversations • Carefully think things through before they speak

(Continued)

Table 9.1   (Continued)

Trait in relation to clinical practice	High level of the trait	Low level of the trait
4. Agreeableness	• Have a great deal of interest in other people • Care about others, especially patients and junior colleagues • Feel empathy and concern for others	• Take little interest in others • Don't care about how others feel even when breaking bad news • Have little interest in other people's problems • Insult and belittle others
5. Neuroticism	• Experience a lot of anxiety, especially in stressful situations • Worry about many different things even if not part of their responsibility • Experience dramatic shifts in mood	• Emotionally stable • Deal well with clinical stress • Rarely feel sad or depressed • Very relaxed

Source: adapted from McCrae and Costa, 1997

BEHAVIOUR THEORY

Behaviour theory focuses on what the leader does, proceeding on specific beliefs about the situation and how the followers function, or are best motivated (see Table 9.2 on leadership styles).

Table 9.2   Leadership styles

Leadership styles	
Theory X and Theory Y (McGregor 1960)	**Theory X:** The central principle of Theory X is direction and control through a centralised system of organisation and the exercise of authority. It is assumed that people are lazy and unmotivated and must be coerced and threatened with punishment if the organisation is to achieve its objective. The average person avoids responsibility, prefers to be directed, lacks ambition and values security. **Theory Y:** Work is seen as natural, like play or rest, and it is assumed that people will exercise self-direction and self-control in the service of objectives to which they are committed. Given the right conditions the average worker can learn to accept and to seek responsibility. Work itself is seen as motivating and rewarding and the environment itself key to motivation.

Leadership styles

Contingency Approach (Fiedler 1967)	**Effective leaders:** will adapt their style and behaviour to the environment, the task, the situation and the people.
Trait Theory of Leadership	**Leadership style** considers that leaders can be chosen for the traits they possess in varying quantities.
	Emergent traits include intelligence and the ability to problem-solve; initiative, independence and inventiveness; self-assurance and self-confidence.
Situational Leadership (Hersey and Blanchard 1969)	**This style of leadership** supports growth and development of team members. There is no single best fit and the style is defined by followers' needs. There are four styles:
	Directing – giving clear instructions.
	Coaching – giving lessons or teaching team members 'on the job'.
	Supporting – facilitating subordinates to sustain the situation.
	Delegating – sharing the task required to care for the patient and their family.
Action Centred Leadership (Adair 1973)	The effective leader must:
	Achieve the task
	Develop the individual
	Build and maintain the team
	Takes account of variables, including leader preferred style, follower preferred style, task and environment
Integrated Leader (Gardner 1990)	Leaders can:
	Think long term, decisions made are not just appropriate for the present, but for the years to come.
	Look outward to the larger organisation, they can see how their clinical setting fits into the larger organisation.
	Influence others beyond their own group, they are effective at working and leading in a multi-professional team.
	Emphasise vision, values and motivation, while upholding their own professional values they are sensitive to other people's values and motivations.
	Be politically astute, they can work within the expectations and conflicts which occur across the organisation and beyond.
	Think in terms of change and renewal, they can remain current within the ever-changing world and work within the organisation to revise practice.

Source: adapted from Thurston, 2013 and Marquis and Huston, 2017

Another behaviour-focused theory often referred to is that of White and Lippitt (1960), which features several quite different styles (see Table 9.3). This theory is useful in allowing the nurse to embrace very different responses depending on the requirements of various situations. The intention is not for these styles to be adopted on a permanent basis but alternated.

Table 9.3   Types of leader

Types of leader	Positive characteristics	Negative characteristics
Autocratic Leader	Quick decision making and implementation of any plan or strategy, works very well in an emergency.	Most of the decisions are made based on the leader's personal opinions, ideas, knowledge, and personality. This can lead to staff disaffection and disempowerment. One negative outcome could be high staff turnover.
Paternalistic Leader	Team members are given utmost priority. But like a parent, the manager may have the final say on all matters. He/she always has the junior team members' best interests in mind.	Team members may become too dependent on their leaders and they are no longer able to use their ideas and creativity to get things done. One negative outcome may be that junior staff will not take decisive actions in clinical emergency situations and could place patients at risk.
Democratic Leader	Open communication occurs on both sides, which in turn may result in better job performance and increased productivity.	It can make decision making slower because it will take longer before people will reach a consensus during discussions and meetings. One negative outcome may be that delays occur in treatment which should have been immediate.
Laissez-faire Leader	With this style, the leader may empower the team and give them the freedom to carry out their tasks, as they deem fit.	It relieves the leader of their duties, which can eventually lead to a lack of coordination and delegation. There may be unsafe practice in the clinical setting and no support for junior members of staff.

Types of leader	Positive characteristics	Negative characteristics
Leadership by Walking Around	Leaders are tasked to 'walk around' and talk to their junior team members on a regular basis. Their objective is to listen to employees' concerns and suggestions, and to foster good working relationships with them.	If carried out by an untrained leader, it could lead to problems especially when they become overly critical of the team. A negative outcome of this could be that staff feel under excessive scrutiny and become unwilling to take any actions without permission.

Source: adapted from http://typesofmanagement.com

Among the more modern theories of leadership are the transactional and democratic. **Transactional leadership** sets targets, and rewards those who meet them and succeed and punishes those who do not. This approach may involve rewarding activity which produces success in meeting the agreed goal. However, a disadvantage is that transactional leadership is dependent on the outcome of the activity. If there is failure, then it may be felt that effort has been overlooked even if this is considerable, and this is a crude and insensitive form of leadership which does not recognise other criteria.

Transformational leadership aims to produce success by:

- Inspiring a shared vision.
- Modelling the way and following preferred standards and offering supervision.
- Being willing to question established protocol.
- Promoting hope, optimism and support.
- Empowering staff to be involved and to feel empowered while promoting self-development.

(Kouzes and Posner 2014)

In contrast with transactional leadership transformational leadership is concerned with the process as opposed to the outcome and includes and actively involves and empowers staff. A disadvantage is that the criteria for success may be ambiguous and much effort is invested in the process of delivering care yet less on identifying whether the outcomes are positive.

Therefore, when considering leadership, it is necessary to think about the attributes of the leader, and the specific circumstances in which this occurs. Stanley and Stanley (2017) draw a useful distinction between leadership and clinical leadership. Clinical leadership refers to, and is inextricably linked to, specific attributes, and therefore is more specific and identifiable in practice.

Clinical leaders are in a non-hierarchical role, and in nursing engage directly with patient care (Cook 2001; Stanley 2006, 2017). Nurses lead through continually improving patient care, which is apparent in their direct actions but also by influencing the work and actions of other staff (Cook 2001). In this respect they act as role models through setting standards by what they do, inspiring others, yet these actions also reflect their values (Stanley and Stanley 2017). Chavez and Yoder (2014: 90) emphasise this point, stating that:

> [staff nurse clinical leadership] is defined as staff nurses who exert significant influence over other individuals in the healthcare team, and although no formal authority has been vested in them, facilitates individual and collective efforts to accomplish shared clinical objectives.

Consistent with this notion, nursing leadership can be understood as a set of discrete and specific attributes, which on their own may seem to be innocuous but if practised in combination create an inclusive environment that is conducive to effective team-working and the delivery of good patient care. Increasingly within nursing, leadership is regarded as being reflected in the range of competencies, skills and aspects of practice with which the nurse is involved (Willis Commission 2012). These include:

- Organising care
- Communicating with colleagues
- Motivating colleagues and staff
- Effective task allocation and delegation
- Promoting team-working
- Supporting staff and colleagues
- Technical skill
- Ability to problem solve
- Coaching colleagues and junior staff.

This renders leadership less of an elusive and mystical set of charismatic skills and characteristics possessed by a few gifted individuals but instead as more reminiscent of situational and transformational leadership, focusing on using team-work and adapting leadership style to suit the relevant situation. Through clinical leadership we can identify a discrete set of competencies and capabilities, which student nurses can embrace as professional values and encourage, promote and foster in teams within which they work and then come to lead.

LEADERSHIP AND MANAGEMENT

The distinction between leadership and management is much discussed (Marquis and Huston 2017; Marriner Tomey 2009; Parkin 2009; Roussel et al. 2009; Sullivan and Decker 2009). However, essentially managers are in a formally appointed role and have legitimate authority with specific goals, outcomes and targets which they are tasked with achieving. The words used to describe the function of management reflect the goal-directed, target-driven nature of this endeavour. Managers are described as having an assigned position in the organisation, including controlling the work and direction of efforts of their team (Marquis and Huston 2017). They work towards defined and specific goals, setting goals and timelines and being responsible for initiating changes and service developments. In contrast, leaders have no formal legitimacy supporting their authority, and often direct willing followers. They obtain power through influence, focusing on group process with an emphasis on interpersonal relationships (Marquis and Huston 2017). Often, they are visionary in approach and work innovatively to inspire and develop others.

Management

Caring for patients and clients can be rewarding but can also be demanding in terms of balancing time, priorities and resources. This requires a range of skills and competencies which include observing, problem-solving, planning and evaluation of clinical actions to ensure the individual receives the most appropriate, evidenced-based care. Nurses work through a range of clinical tasks during any given day to facilitate a well-organised holistic approach to care. Through experience you will have learned from role models, reading and reflection that there are many ways of dealing with situations. You will develop your own style or way of dealing with situations.

This section of the chapter will enable students from all fields of nursing to develop skills in management supporting the transition from student to registered practitioner, leading a team of nurses. This transition involves adjusting to a new and challenging role, accepting changing responsibilities and developing further complex skills that allow the effective management of care as well as its delivery. Several high-profile reports have highlighted the important link between effective leadership and management in nursing and patient experience and outcome (Berwick 2013; Francis 2013; Keogh 2013). This transition provides students with the opportunity to act as a leader, coach, supporter and supervisor for junior students and colleagues (Willis 2012). It also involves promoting students' growth and expertise in professional knowledge, judgement and self-awareness (Keogh 2013).

Risk assessment and management are equally as important in supporting patient safety, and as students you should have had the opportunity to consider how patient safety may be enhanced through an exploration of human factors and system design. Practice competencies form the basis for development and assessment in the practice setting. These competencies should be demonstrated to provide safe and autonomous practice to be successful as a qualified nurse, see **Chapters 6 and 7** on fitness to practice and clinical governance and delegation.

The process of management is a personal undertaking which suggests that every individual manager will manage staff differently, because all managers are humans and all individuals are unique. As individual nurses you have unique thoughts about your roles and responsibilities, which includes your own set of values, derived from your personality, work and life experiences; every person will think and act in a way that captures this. While knowing theories, philosophies and protocols is a very important part of managing teams, it is vital to remember that teams are made up of these unique individuals. The group therefore is not homogenised; rather each person brings with them both strengths and areas for development. A rule or policy may work for the majority but not for everyone. (See Michael Coffey [2018] and his teachings on management at Anglia Ruskin University.)

There is a balance between ensuring patient safety and ensuring staff are satisfied in their roles; this means that there are areas of practice where flexibility cannot be adopted, such as routines for prescribed medications and treatments which must be maintained for patient safety. However, other areas, such as the ward rota, holidays, etc., should feel more like a democratic process. You cannot manage a team by numbers or formulas. As a manager you need to have self-awareness about yourself and what you expect from the team members. The process begins by acknowledging what management of a clinical setting requires, and the factors which may affect this. The roles of a manager in clinical practice include:

- **Planning** – including organising routine activities, such as stores, even when not physically present.
- **Staffing** – including ensuring an appropriate skills mix and staff rotas.
- **Organising** – including which staff members work in each team, and how the nursing teams work with the interprofessional team.
- **Reporting** – including compiling both internal reports to hospital managers such as bed numbers and clinical audits and the external reports for CQC or NMC, when requested.
- **Budgeting** – one of the most challenging elements of managing a clinical or community environment, to ensure you have enough resources for the predicted workload being undertaken throughout the year (see Table 9.4).
- **Coordinating** – this includes working with the MDT and the rest of the health Trust to ensure that outcomes are achieved. This could be as simple as food arriving at meal times or medication deliveries, or more complex issues such as rehabilitation or hours in casualty.
- **Directing** – you cannot undertake all the managing by yourself, as services are often 24/7 and the ward manager works 37 hours a week. Therefore there is a requirement to direct and support the individuals left in charge when you are not present.

Management is undertaken using different types of skills including technical, human and conceptual.

- **Technical skills**
  - Important, particularly for individuals in lower management roles, to perform work based tasks, linked closely to overall productivity and coalface working with colleagues

- **Human skills**
  - These skills are needed for all levels of management; it is important to have the ability to work with individuals and groups
- **Conceptual skills**
  - This is of substantial importance, particularly for top management. There is a requirement to be able to see abstract and sometimes complicated ideas especially across a whole organisation

(Adapted from Katz 1974, 2009)

It is also important to get to know the different types of management approaches and skills and how your own personal insights help you become a good manager. Knowing the different types of management can help you determine which type or style would suit you best, based on your own skills, personality and abilities, as well as other factors such as the kind of people you will be handling and your clinical work environment.

Often there are a mixture of styles depending on the situation and the professionals you are working with. If you have self-awareness you can change the way you manage, both in small ways, such as letting staff decide on meal breaks and in more significant ways, such as planning the requirements needed for 24-hour care. Some of this may relate to trusting the team and the individual, but it also needs to be remembered that every member of qualified staff must work within their code of conduct.

The starting point for this is to understand what management is and is not and to establish the key issues affecting clinical practice regarding leadership of the area. The people you manage need to do the things for which you have overall accountability. As a manager, you do not perform productive work alone; the people who work for you perform most of the hands-on skills. Indeed, this principle is often used as the litmus test of whether you are managing or doing: if you are doing the work you are not managing. As managers you must seamlessly move between the routine and typical, and the one-off or emergency situation. Because of this there needs to be an openness to new approaches and input from others, and you need to empower team members to voice their opinion and develop through the process. The personal attributes and the ability to communicate beliefs and values in the manager role is as important as the skills to undertake technical and clinical tasks. Without appropriate communication you will not be able to understand, respect and have confidence in the team's relationships.

Due to movement of staff, skill-mix can change and new priorities will become evident. It is at this point where personal development plans may indicate staff with interests for further development. This fits with the notion of lifelong learning and evidenced-based practice (NMC 2014). The individual's performance at work can be determined by the extrinsic rewards (external rewards for example salary and status) and the intrinsic rewards (internal rewards like self-recognition and worthwhileness).

Table 9.4 Management of resources

Resource	Examples	Requirements	Risks
Physical Resources	Purchasing equipment can vary from weekly (such as needles, syringes) to the 'big purchases' (hoists, profiling beds).	All equipment should be fit for purpose and well maintained. Mandatory training programmes and records. Tracking equipment from serial numbers is important.	Systems breakdown. Staff taking shortcuts. Communication breakdown. Ill-defined responsibility. Poor training systems. Poor coordination of equipment records, maintenance and repairs.
Financial Resources	Budget management can be set at either ward level with the ward manager, or with a group of wards at matron/lead nurse level or at the higher level of the most senior nurse in directorate/division.	Stock control. Sharing resources with others.	No coordination on buying resources. Lack of stock control. Inadequate researching of products leading to more expensive material. High levels of wastage.
Human Resources	Staffing accounts for the largest proportion of the NHS budget. This requires strategic planning and is reviewed when there is a change to the specific clinical area.	Investment in staff development. Requirements for an area known as the 'establishment'. Number of types of staff and their grades which are required to ensure the safe and effective running of the specific clinical area.	Confusing collection of tools which calculate the number of nurses required to care for an estimated acuity of patients within a setting. Some of these tools have been based on time and motion studies. Some have been based on task and time requirements and others on 'multipliers'. During winter pressures or during acute, high-dependency admissions the need may arise to adjust the usual nursing establishment of staff in the clinical environment.

Source: adapted from Thurston, 2013

Time management

As you become more confident in your practice and have higher levels of motivation, your time management skills become more honed. Time is a precious commodity and poor time management has an impact on costs of service delivery (Huber 2010). Care interventions can be planned across the shift pattern rather than condensing it all into a few hours. You need to consider building in time management strategies to deal with any emergency or unplanned situation as they are presented. A few moments checking the functionality of oxygen and suction supplies at the beginning of a shift could save valuable seconds if faced with a resuscitation situation. In the community it may be that you check that you have everything required for the group of patients or clients you are visiting, including equipment, phone numbers and documentation. Routine practice has been debated within the nursing press with supporters and critics. Without advocating a return to the situation where ritualistic nursing practice is the order of the day, it would seem a sensible option that provided the routine practice had an evidence basis and a substantial part of a patient's care is individualised, the two concepts both have a place in contemporary nursing (Thurston 2013).

REFERENCES

Adair, J., (1973). *Action-Centred Leadership*. London: McGraw-Hill.

Berwick Report (2013). *A Promise to Learn – a Commitment to Act: Improving the Safety of Patients in England*. National Advisory Group on the Safety of Patients in England. London: Crown Publishing.

Chavez, E.C. and Yoder, L.H. (2014). Staff nurse clinical leadership: a concept analysis. *Nursing Forum*, 50(2): 90–100.

Coffey, M. (2018). Management Theory module, Anglia Ruskin University. *Lecture notes* 2018.

Cook, M.J. (2001). The attributes of effective clinical nurse leaders. *Nursing Standard*, 15(35): 33–6.

Fiedler (1967). *A Theory of Leadership Effectiveness*. New York: McGraw-Hill.

Francis, R. (2013). *Report of the Mid Staffordshire NHS Foundation Trust Public Inquiry*. London: The Stationery Office.

Gardner, J. W. (1990). *On Leadership*. New York, NY: Free Press.

Hersey, P., and Blanchard, K.H. (1969). Life cycle theory of leadership. *Training and Development Journal*, 23(2), 26–34.

Huber, D. (2010). *Leadership and Nursing Care Management*. St Louis, MO: Elsevier Saunders.

Katz, R.L. (1974). Skills of an effective administrator. *Harvard Business Review*. Republished 2009 by Harvard Business School Publishing Corporation.

Keogh Report (2013). Review into the Quality of Care and Treatment Provided by 14 Hospital Trusts in England: Overview Report. Professor Sir Bruce Keogh KBE.

Kouzes, J.M. and Posner, B.Z. (2014). *The Five Practices of Exemplary Leadership*, 2nd ed. San-Francisco: Pfeffer.

Marquis, B.L. and Huston, C.J. (2017). *Leadership Roles and Management Functions in Nursing: Theory and Application*, 9th ed. Philadelphia: Wolters Kluwer.

Marriner Tomey, A. (2009). *Guide to Nursing Management and Leadership*, 8th ed. St Louis, MO: Elsevier Mosby.

McCrae, R.R. and Costa, P.T. (1997). Personality trait structure as a human universal. *American Psychologist*, 52: 509–16.

McGregor, Douglas M. (1960). *The Human Side of Enterprise*. New York: McGraw-Hill.

NHS (2015). *The NHS Constitution: The NHS Belongs to Us All*. https://assets.publishing. service.gov.uk/government/uploads/system/uploads/attachment_data/file/480482/ NHS_Constitution_WEB.pdf. London: Crown Copyright.

Northouse, P.G. (2018). *Leadership: Theory and Practice*. London: Sage.

Nursing and Midwifery Council (NMC) (2014). Standards for competence for registered nurses. www.nmc.org.uk/globalassets/sitedocuments/standards/nmc-standards-for-competence-for-registered-nurses.pdf

Parkin, P. (2009). *Managing Change in Healthcare: Using Action Research*. London: Sage.

Pepin, J., Dubois, S., Girard, F., Tardif, J. and Ha, L. (2010). A cognitive learning model of clinical nursing leadership. *Nurse Education Today*, 31: 268–73.

Roussel, L., Swansburg, R.C. and Swansburg, R.J. (eds) (2009). *Management and Leadership for Nurse Administrators*, 5th ed. Burlington, MA: Jones and Bartlett Publishers.

Stanley, D. (2006). In command of care: toward the theory of congruent leadership. *Journal of Research in Nursing*, 11(2), 132–44.

Stanley, D. (2017). *Clinical Leadership in Nursing and Healthcare: Values into Action*. Oxford: Wiley-Blackwell.

Stanley, D. and Stanley, K. (2017). Clinical leadership and nursing explored: a literature search. *Journal of Clinical Nursing*, 27: 1730–43.

Sullivan, E.J. and Decker, P.J. (2009). *Effective Leadership and Management in Nursing*, 7th ed. London: Prentice Hall.

Sullivan, E.J. and Garland, G. (2010). *Practical Leadership and Management in Nursing*. Harlow: Pearson

Thurston, C. (ed.) (2013). *Essential Nursing Care for Children and Young People*. London: Routledge.

Types of Management (n.d.). http://typesofmanagement.com/

White, R.K. and Lippitt, R. (1960). *Autocracy and Democracy: An Experimental Enquiry*. New York: Harper & Row.

Whitehead, D.K., Weiss, S.A. and Tappen, R.M. (2010). *Essentials of Nursing Leadership and Management*, 5th ed. Philadelphia: F.A. Davis Company.

Willis Commission (2012). *Quality with Compassion: The Future of Nursing Education*. Published by the Royal College of Nursing on behalf of the independent Willis Commission on Nursing Education.

10

Conclusion

Resilience and compassion in qualified practice

Nick Wrycraft

'A human being is a spatially and temporally limited piece of the whole, what we call the "Universe." He experiences himself and his feelings as separate from the rest, an optical illusion of his consciousness. The quest for liberation from this bondage is the only object of true religion. Not nurturing the illusion but only overcoming it gives us the attainable measure of inner peace.'

(Albert Einstein)

This chapter covers similar factors to **Chapter 1**, albeit from a different perspective, consistent with the theme of this book of transitions. While Chapter 1 focused on developing from being a third-year student to becoming a qualified nurse, in contrast this chapter considers the transition challenges I experienced in the early stages of my career.

Learning outcomes

- The transition from being a newly qualified to experienced nurse.
- The challenges we may undergo during this process.
- Reflecting on the changes that occur as a result.

We begin the discussion by considering the transition to becoming a newly qualified nurse, and the experience of impostor phenomena, before addressing a range of factors that are commonly relevant involved in transitions. These include: **Age, Self, Personality, Intelligence, Education, Environment, Family and Society**.

TRANSITION PROGRESS

Qualifying as a nurse represents a milestone in your career, and a huge achievement. Inevitably during the three years or more of study that you have undertaken there will have been personal trials and challenges, and the nature of these differs for everyone. If at a particularly low moment or moments, you have not thought of leaving the course at least once then there is something amiss. Revisiting our reason(s) for wanting to become a nurse helps to reaffirm our core motivation. For a few the cost may exceed the benefit, and they may end their studies, but for others this process cements their resolve and provides them with increased certainty as to their choice of career. For me resolve and commitment has been reinforced through my career by seeing what I believed being affirmed in the commitment and skills of other nurses, and is reaffirmed in seeing the commitment of the nurses of the future in my current work in nurse education. Perhaps I have become more of a nurse by being a nurse. I would prefer to think that the fulfilment I have gained from my role has increased my commitment.

Activity 10.1

Think of an occasion when you contemplated leaving the course.

- Consider the circumstances that triggered these doubts.
- Now reflect on what led you to continue.
- Compare this with the reason(s) why you joined the course, and see if they are the same.
- Write the explanation(s) of why you stayed on the course down.
- Now read it.
- On reviewing this it may be the case that this explanation seems simple and helps to make sense of sometimes complicated feelings.

Often the reason(s) people want to become a nurse is a powerful and enduring motivation. It may be the experience of seeing a loved one, or close family member receiving excellent care. Alternatively, it may be that you had a relative with an ongoing health issue. Or even that you have received or witnessed poor care and want to improve the patient experience. Often students say they want to make a difference, which echoes the title of a well-known Department of Health publication from a long while ago but the dominant sentiments have an enduring relevance:

> Nurses, midwives and health visitors are vital to the NHS, and to the nation: they make a real difference to people's lives. People trust them, and have confidence in them ...

> (DoH 1999: 4)

It is important to retain an awareness of your reasons for joining the profession so that there is a consistent thread and focus to your experience, and you can keep hold of who you are, and why you are a nurse when experiencing doubts, as this will sustain you in the future.

In the early days of post-qualified practice, it is not unusual to feel overwhelmed, unequal to the task, or even unworthy of the role. Peternelli-Taylor (2011) discusses Clance and Imes's (1978) work on **impostor phenomena** where the person in a position of responsibility undergoes immense self-doubt and uncertainty and experiences concerns that they will be revealed as a fraud and incapable, even where they are perfectly well qualified. The person may be aware that they have achieved qualified status, yet still undergo these feelings. Impostor phenomena are frequently experienced by people who tend to have exacting demands of themselves and compare themselves to others.

Impostor phenomena seem to be especially relevant to nursing. Often as a newly qualified nurse you may be working alongside other colleagues who are vastly experienced and with high levels of expertise. In this situation you may set high expectations of your own performance, against which you can only fall short. From my own experience impostor phenomena wore off but took around eighteen months to do so. However, feeling these doubts can be immensely anxiety provoking and troubling. I found it helpful to talk to other newly qualified nurses and to trusted colleagues and my preceptor.

EXPLORATION OF FACTORS

Age

Through life we undergo a series of events that mark major transitions or milestones as we develop and grow. These include completing your compulsory education and receiving the right to vote and being entered on the electoral register. Yet in themselves these transitions do not represent an achievement, as we do not need to do anything to gain these benefits. It has been noted that in societies where there is a high level of mutual dependence and close societal bonds transitions are often marked by 'rites of passage'. Commonly this takes the form of a trial or ordeal, related to some activity that has significance to the cultural identity of the group. Often 'rites of passage' is taken as referring to whole societies, yet it can also refer to sub-groups within a wider population and to use two examples related to health, in terms of providers and consumers, this can be applied to surgeons for example (Veazey Brooks and Bosk 2012); or people who undergo cosmetic surgery on a frequent basis (Schouten 1991), or any group of people bound together by an element of common identity. Often the nature of the act or challenge of the rite of passage is connected to the factors that bind the individuals together, and in this way, there is a deep sense of trust. The successful completion of the trial leads to the person being accepted and gaining in status and prestige. While rites of passage contribute to societal cohesion and serve to imbue a sense of shared meaning and identity, a disadvantage is that this form of social organisation reinforces hierarchy, and can lead to individuals who have other skill sets than those that are tested being ostracised or unvalued by the community.

Within our cosmopolitan culture there are few clear stages or points of transition and a disadvantage of this is that individuals can experience a sense of flux, confusion or loss of identity and not feeling as though they belong, have a role, or can contribute meaningfully to the community. Erik Erikson (1902–1994) identified a crucial number of key stages in our life and development and specific challenges relevant to each, which we need to successfully negotiate in order to progress to the next stage (Table 10.1). Failure to effectively overcome the challenge at a certain stage can inhibit the individual's development and progression to maturity. Therefore, while the person may physically grow and age, psychosocially their development may be stifled.

Table 10.1   Erikson's life stages

Psychosocial crisis	Virtue	Age
Trust vs Mistrust	Hope	Infancy (0–1½)
Autonomy vs Shame	Will	Early childhood (1½–3)
Initiative vs Guilt	Purpose	Play Age (3–5)
Industry vs Inferiority	Competency	School Age (5–12)
Ego Identity vs Role Confusion	Fidelity	Adolescence (12–18)
Intimacy vs Isolation	Love	Young Adulthood (18–40)
Generativity vs Stagnation	Care	Adulthood (40–65)
Ego Integrity vs Despair	Wisdom	Maturity (65+)

Source: Erikson 1968

Erikson's original eighth stage referred to people in their 80s. However, over the course of the latter part of the twentieth century internationally there has been a consistent and growing trend of people living significantly longer than in previous eras. Therefore Joan Erikson who was married to Erik Erikson also suggested a ninth stage, relevant to people in the older stage of old age (Erikson 1998).

Quite touchingly she drew these observations from her own experience of ageing and seeing Erikson himself age. She conceptualises that this stage was relevant to people in their late 80s and 90s, and was in her 90s herself when she wrote about this stage (Brown and Lowis 2003). The challenge experienced at the ninth stage was to revisit all of the previous eight stages with the order of the stages being reversed, so that for the first stage the dilemma is of Mistrust vs Trust. There is evidence to support Joan Erikson's notion that we continue to change and develop even in later life. In explaining these findings, Johnson and Barer (1993) in a study of 150 individuals aged 85 and older found that people adapted to physical and social loss through adopting coping mechanisms that focus on specific problems, and living in the present, even though they were declining in functioning. Therefore, consistent with Joan Erikson's theory Johnson and Barer (1993) suggest that we continue to develop even towards the end of life through changing our time orientation from the future to the present and reconciling ourselves to our own mortality. This may be seen as contradicting Joan Erikson's notion that in the ninth stage we revisit all of the stages of our earlier challenges and is consistent with Heidegger's (2003) notion of how we exist within time, as only being within the present. Heidegger (2003) in characteristically idiosyncratic language speaks of us as being 'thrown' into the world, and espouses an existentialist view wherein we live within the present, and can only be aware of the here and now. I feel though that we represent the entirety of our past in the here and now. We are the product of our own narrative story so far, and this means that we will all have a different perspective predicated by the life that we have lived until now. I feel that the power of reminiscence and reliving and reviewing our past from the vantage point of ourselves at a later point in life is in itself something rewarding.

Look at Erikson's life stage model in Table 10.1. Identify the stage you are on in Erikson's life stage model, and reflect as to whether the pertinent crisis is something that is relevant for you at the moment.

Activity 10.2

Self

Our notion of self and identity is crucial to the professionals we become. How we understand who we are, and the beliefs that we have about how the self is constructed and exists within society is not simply an act of introspection but has valuable benefits. The philosophy that we have about the self has significant consequences in determining how we are when working with the patients for whom we care, yet also in determining how we work with colleagues, how we set priorities, and our beliefs about health, health care and the role and function of nursing.

The nature of our self is influenced by our innate nature, the influential figures in our lives, such as parents, carers, guardians, relatives, our social network and the society in which we live. In addition to this the experiences we undergo contributes towards shaping the self that we become. Developmental theorists unanimously suggest that we are largely formed in our youth and that after these early stages of being moulded, we change only to a limited extent, unless an exceptional event or trauma occurs to fundamentally change our nature (Bowlby 1997, 1998a, 1998b; Erikson 1968; Piaget 2000).

Our self is the person that we are in the present. Yet we know ourselves through how we appear to others, and the feedback that we receive, both direct and indirect. Often the self is therefore evident through a process of mediation. We make choices of how to act as personal decisions in how we behave and the manner in which we interact and communicate with others. Yet we also make decisions based on how we want to be perceived by others. Some people are very autonomous and self-determining, while others are highly influenced by the social environment, and want to be accepted. Julian Rotter (1966) developed the locus of control theory. Those with a high level of internal locus of control believe that they can determine and influence outcomes, while those with a high external locus of control believe that they are less directly influential and more dependent upon external circumstances. The locus of control is often referred to with regard to health related behaviour and help seeking.

Some working roles require a high level of investment of the self, and others more conformity to a uniform identity depending on the nature of the role. In nursing, where there is close working alongside other nurses and professionals, acquiring a sense of belonging and feeling part of and accepted within a working community is important in the development of students' identity as a nurse (Levett-Jones and Lathlean 2008). Walker et al. (2014) carried out research into the elements that contribute to student nurses' developing identity while on clinical placement, and among other aspects found acceptance to be central in a positive learning experience, as the following comment illustrates:

> The ward was very welcoming; my name was placed on the patient allocation list each shift which gave me some autonomy and sense of belonging. The staff thanked me each shift for my help, which gave me a sense of worthiness, and often included me in conversations about the work environment and social occasions, which boosted my confidence and also made me feel like a team member.
>
> (Walker et al. 2014: 107)

As this quote demonstrates, small acts of consideration and inclusion can produce a significant impact on the perception, confidence and attitude of students. Conversely, students' feelings of acceptance can be undermined by the absence of certain elements, such as:

> lack of direction, limited learning opportunities, and poor communication between ward staff, facility management and the tertiary teaching facilities responsible for arranging clinical placements.
>
> (Walker et al. 2014: 107)

The findings of this study indicate that the learning environment has a significant impact on the identity of student nurses. It is worth considering though how our identity as professionals continues to be influenced and shaped as we progress as qualified professionals responsible for our own practice but under preceptorship and then as an autonomous professional. The nature of nurse education and promotion of lifelong learning emphasises that we continue to learn throughout our career, and our identity continues to form and adapt.

Consider whether you are a person who is very self-determining, or requires a high level of social acceptance.

Can you identify instances or examples where you have demonstrated this behaviour?

Do you feel a need to become more autonomous or to seek greater social acceptance?

What steps might you take to achieve this goal?

How will you know that this goal has been achieved?

Activity 10.3

Author's own experience

As a student nurse I felt vulnerable going to new placements but was met with a warm, welcoming and supportive response, and I felt accepted and respected. It surprised me how the staff did not use rank or position but accepted me as an equal. The openness, honesty and willingness to express their views, and even ask my opinion was something I respected and admired about the qualified nurses. There was an awareness of the weight of accountability, but also and as a consequence, a commitment towards using this to advocate on behalf of people with mental health issues. Even though there were varied approaches to practice, with some senior nurses more autocratic than others, I felt that my colleagues valued me. Within teams there was an active awareness and cultivation of team support and looking out, yet not covering, for one another. The sense of belonging I gained is something that I still feel today, and value. When I meet people with whom I worked, even many years ago there is an instant sense of rapport and understanding, no matter how much time has elapsed since we last met. On reflection I have often lacked a sense of belonging and identity in my life. I think I found a sense of acceptance and belonging.

Personality

While the self identifies the proximity or extent to which I exert control over my behavioural and communication choices and how I stand in my relationship with others, personality refers to the content and finer detail of what constitutes the nature of these exchanges. Personality offers a finer and more detailed description of who we are. It can be understood as the individual behavioural, emotional and thought processes in which we engage (Hakamata and Inada 2011). Often personality is thought of as being composed of traits or dispositions that can be measured, and although there has been significant work and research there is no definitive consensus on what these are (Allport and Odbert 1936; Cattell 1943; Fiske 1949). More recent research though suggests that the structure of the brain determines qualities within personality (Celikel 2011). One theory suggested by Cloninger et al. (1994), based upon the connections between personality and neurobiology, suggests that there are seven factors, four of which pertain to temperament (harm avoidance, novelty seeking, reward dependence and persistence) and three to character (self-directedness, cooperativeness and self-transcendence). Temperament is the emotional centre of personality (Celikel 2011; Cloninger et al. 1994); it refers to our tendency towards emotions such as fear, anger and attachment and can be observed in infancy, and is genetically determined, remaining stable across the lifespan (Svrakic et al. 2002; Whittle et al. 2006). In contrast, character refers to cognitive processes such as logical thought, interpreting the meaning of symbols and skills of invention. These aspects are thought to be influenced to some extent by family relationships and change over time and as we gain in maturity (Celikel 2011). Broadly consistent with the notion of personality as being comprised of temperament and feelings, character represents more logical aspects. Cognitive Behavioural Therapy (CBT) views the self as composed of four aspects. These are: thoughts, mood, behaviour and physiology (Greenberger and Padesky 1995; Skinner and Wrycraft 2014). In CBT the practitioner uses this model to identify where the harmony between these elements may be out of balance, which might indicate areas of their life where the patient may be experiencing difficulties.

Activity 10.4

Consider whether you are more a feelings or thought-led person?

Reflect on how this influences you in practice.

Consider how you might develop aspects of yourself to become more the practitioner you want to be.

Author's own experience

The greatest hurdle for me in learning to be a nurse, even long into post-registration, has been engaging the feelings part of myself in my work and permitting myself to be 'my-self' at work. As a person I struggle to show my feelings at times, and have often been reserved, and reluctant to show how I feel. When working on an adult acute mental health unit, I often admired how other qualified nurses were able to disclose to other nurses how they felt about their work. Some years later, when carrying out my Doctoral research into group clinical supervision with community based practitioners, I was again vividly impressed by how nurses and other health professionals were very open about their feelings and expressed anger, guilt, resentment and shame in relation to their work. Over time I have become better at being my-self, and it has surprised me how this is helpful and uses up less emotional energy than being controlled all of the time. I feel that this is consistent with my personality, as I value integrity. At the same time, in terms of tempera- ment, being honest about my feelings acknowledges how they affect me, and this has allowed me to be my-self, and I have felt much more able to be more open about my work and my feelings about my work. Martin Heidegger (2003) talked about the notion of authenticity and being who we are. In his philosophy Heidegger intended the term to have a more technical and complex application, but essentially authen- ticity has some meaning in this context. Being who we are, and true to ourselves, could be argued to be essential for our emotional and psy- chological wellbeing, yet also for our fulfilment and sense of belonging in the world and for our identity as nurses.

Intelligence

Often intelligence is regarded as being related to problem solving or complex cognitive skills and rational thought. Within nursing though a significant amount of time is spent working with and alongside other health care professionals and patients, their families and significant others, which inevitably involves significant exposure to people undergoing stress and distress. Inevitably this has an impact and requires the application of skills in order to be able to successfully adapt and manage in practice without this having an effect upon the nurse's physical and mental wellbeing and health. In 1983 Hochschild identified the term 'emotional labour', to reflect how workers adapt their feelings and manage their responses when working with people in accordance with social norms and rules within the workplace (Delgado et al. 2017). Within this theory, in order to conform to workplace norms, workers engage in deep acting or surface acting. Deep acting is where the person induces real or genuine emotion, whereas surface acting is where the person simulates an unfelt emotion or suppresses their genuine feelings (Hochschild, 2003). Because of the compatibility with the worker's gen- uine feelings, deep acting is associated with job satisfaction and fulfilment. In contrast, surface acting due to the dissonance this represents with the person's true self can lead to inner conflict, stress and dissatisfaction. In relation to nurs- ing three areas have been identified regarding emotional labour. These areas are therapeutic, collegial and instrumental, whereby therapeutic emotion labour is evident in relationships with patients, family and significant others, collegial pertains to relations with other clinicians, and instrumental refers to the nurse's confidence in communication skills and competence performing technical procedures and interventions (Delgado et al. 2017). From conducting a literature review focused on emotional labour in nursing in these domains Delgado et al. (2017) identified under-recognition of the effect of collegial aspects in contributing to nurses' experience of emotional labour. This suggests that the contribution of collegial relations to emotional labour is under-recognised. Delgado et al. (2017) attributed this to the predominantly female composition of the nursing workforce, and gendered attitudes leading to assumptions that this is simply an accepted part of the job.

While the nature of nursing as involving increasingly technical work and close relationships with unwell patients and concerned families and significant others inherently predisposes nurses to experience emotional labour, it should not be regarded as an inevitable consequence. The effects of emotional labour can lead to occupational stress and burnout yet may also be reduced by developing emotional resilience to promote sustainability in nurses (Delgado et al. 2017). Among the solutions to reducing emotional labour within nursing is to enhance leadership training, and a central element to this is developing emotional intelligence including self-compassion. Carragher and Gormley (2017) consider different competing models of emotional intelligence. They identify that there is debate about the authenticity of emotional intelligence, with some dismissing it as a concept at all, or suggesting that rationality and cognitive intelligence may be more suited to guiding leadership decisions. However, Carragher and Gormley (2017) reasonably point out that nursing is grounded in caring and therefore emotional intelligence ought to be a central component of leadership. The evidence base supporting emotional intelligence is equivocal, with little unanimity in even agreeing an overall model. There are three main different models (see Table 10.2).

Table 10.2 Models of emotional intelligence

Model/Author	Features
Ability-Based Model (Mayer et al. 2004)	Four levels of emotional abilities: • Perception of emotion within self and others; • Assimilation of emotion to facilitate thought; • Understanding emotion; • Managing and regulating emotion, in self and others.
Trait-Based Model (Bar-On 2002, 2006)	Emotional intelligence is an aspect of personality which focuses on traits for example: • Empathy • Emotional Expression • Adaptability • Self-Control

Model/Author	Features
Mixed model (Goleman 1995, 1998)	Five skill domains Personal effectiveness: 1. Personal effectiveness 2. Self-awareness 3. Self-regulation and motivation Social competence: 4. Empathy 5. Social skills

Activity 10.5

Look at the above understandings of emotional labour.

Choose one and consider how your profile maps onto the characteristics.

Are there any areas where you need to develop your competence?

Author's own experience

Nursing is an inherently human profession. The nurses I most admired over the years, and who made the biggest impact on me were people whose human qualities were very clearly evident, and who were comfortable engaging with others interpersonally. As a person I am a quiet individual, and sensitive. In the past I have felt that people have identified that in me, and it made me feel vulnerable and sometimes inclined to be defensive. Over time, though, I came to perceive communication as not only being the transmission of information but also expressing need(s). This might be direct, in terms of asking for something, or indirect, or even something of which the person is not aware. For example, I might feel embarrassed at asking for help, and so not specifically ask but hope that this need is recognised, or deliver hints, as opposed to declaring my need explicitly. Therefore, when communicating, if we can understand what the other person wants or needs this avoids conflict, misunderstanding or disappointment. This is especially useful in mental health nursing, where often people struggle to communicate their needs, or express themselves effectively. I feel that I have become more empathic and accepting of people. I try to listen, and not just to the verbal content of what the person is saying but what they really mean. It is easy to understand empathy, but engaging in it and doing it is another thing entirely. Through considering why a person might think or feel how they do, it is much easier to understand them and communicate positively and constructively. That is not to condone poor behaviour when people struggle to communicate and become frustrated, just that if people feel listened to then they are much less likely to become frustrated and angry.

Education

As adult learners the nature of our experience is different than our compulsory education up until the age of eighteen. Knowles (1980) suggests that the way we learn as adults differs from children. While children tend to accept what they are taught unquestioningly, as adults we are autonomous and self-determining in educational experiences. As adult learners we subject information to greater scrutiny and compare and assimilate it to our previous knowledge. This means that we interpret information differently, are more curious and challenging learners, and make decisions about what to prioritise, and what it means. Within Knowles' theory of andragogy there are six aspects that characterise how we learn as we grow and mature (Table 10.3).

Table 10.3   Knowles' theory of andragogy

Aspect	Features
Self-concept	As people mature, we transition from dependence to self-directed learning.
Experience	As adults our experiences provide a fertile resource for learning.
Readiness to learn	As we mature, we become interested in learning subjects with immediate relevance to our jobs or lives.
Orientation to learning	As we grow older our time perspective changes from gathering knowledge for future use to immediate application. Adult learners are problem rather than subject focused.
Motivation to learn	As people mature, they are motivated by internal incentives, such as self-esteem, curiosity, the desire to achieve, and sense of accomplishment.
Relevance	Adult learners need to know why they need to learn something. Furthermore, because adults have other responsibilities, they ought to be involved in planning and implementing learning.

Source: Knowles 1980; Knowles et al. 2005

Within Knowles' theory of andragogy, as adults we approach learning with a pre-existent agenda and set of expectations about the value, purpose and use for the learning that we undergo.

Activity 10.6

Looking at Knowles' theory of andragogy:

- Which are the most important for you, and apply to you as a learner?
- Are there aspects that you had not previously thought about but which capture your attention?
- Are there any aspects which you feel are especially relevant for your role as a nurse?

Author's own experience

At school I was always far more capable at academic subjects. Yet I lacked confidence at practical subjects, and struggled to ask for help, or was self-conscious about my lack of ability, and so did not try. As a result, I concentrated only on certain subjects at the expense of others. I felt I only had a narrow range of capability and lacked confidence at practical subjects. My confidence and willingness to engage with different aspects of knowledge improved though when I began to train as a nurse. This was because nursing represents a wide and disparate body of ideas and information from numerous subjects including biology, law, psychology, sociology, and even and increasingly information technology. I found training to be a nurse as an adult learner was a valuable experience. I was studying for several of the reasons Knowles identifies. On a practical level it was to gain a professional qualification and access a career, yet I found the knowledge to be valuable in itself and empowering in practice. As a student mental health nurse, the history of my profession is controversial and political. However, the heterogeneous nature of nursing also opened up a world of information freed from the narrow confines of specific subjects. As I have grown older, I have also derived a more personal meaning and interpretation of what I learn which spans my professional and personal life. I often revisit concepts and ideas I have studied before, only to gain a new and changed appreciation.

Environment

Often the effects of sociological factors on health and development are overlooked. The Marmot Review (2010) even identified a clear correlation between social situation and mortality, and among the contributing factors to this is the environment in which we live. Environment includes housing and the quality, standard and nature of living conditions, transport, crime and safety. Yet also the accessibility of amenities as well as the natural environment.

What factors have been influential in your development within nursing?

- To what extent have these factors made an impact upon you?
- How situation specific are these?
- Do you feel that other student nurses' environments lead them to have a very different experience?

Activity 10.7

(Continued)

(Continued)

Author's own experience

I grew up and lived for the first 22 years of my life in the same house in a small seaside town. I later worked for the local council as a housing officer in the same area, and then trained as a nurse. The locality was poor, and my family struggled to get by financially. When I worked for the local council I again encountered numerous experiences of poverty and social deprivation. When I trained as a nurse all of my clinical placements were in the town where I had grown up, and when on placement with the community mental health team I visited some of the same patients I had worked with on the inpatient ward. Some of the issues that fed into the experience of people with ongoing issues were the same as I had witnessed when working in housing.

I also happened to be training at the same time as the most momentous change in decades, with the dismantling of the large institutions, and mental health services being dispersed and re-provisioned in the community. On placement, I found a strong common and shared culture among the staff who had all worked together in the same institution in very recent memory. There was a sense of duty but also feelings of abandonment and loss, and perhaps even also resentment that such a radical change was being imposed as the institution had existed for nearly a century and the staff clung on to aspects of their former identity. For example, a ward that was relocated from the institution took all of the dining room furniture, the ward clock and even some clinical supplies that were past their use-by date.

Family

Even though we live in an increasingly fragmented society, relationships with close significant others, parents, partners and siblings are still fundamental, not only in moulding who we are but providing us with a sense of direction, feeling of inclusion and purpose in life. Influential development theorists such as Bowlby (1997, 1998a, 1998b), Erikson (1968) and Piaget (2000) all suggest that our identity and who we are is largely shaped over a brief period of successive stages when we are children and young people. While we may change and develop later in life these are for the most part less radical and more gradual and incremental changes. Yet undergoing a major life change and development through becoming a nurse inevitably makes an impact on who we are and has the potential to change relationships within families.

How have your family responded to you training to become a nurse?

- Have your family relationships changed during your time training to become a nurse?
- What has contributed to these changes?

Author's own experience

My father and a number of the men in my family are carpenters, and from a young age I used to work with and help him even up until my late teens. I always assumed I would follow this line of work. However, I found it difficult, and did not have a natural affinity for carpentry. After leaving university I worked for several years as a housing officer. The job had no prospects, and in the end, I realised that a change was necessary. My mother was an adult nurse and underwent her training when I was between the ages of 8 and 11. I was proud of her, and during her career she became a charge nurse, managed several wards, and was well respected as a leader who always supported her staff. I was not sure I had the necessary skills to do this work, and have always been more interested in psychosocial aspects of people than their physical functioning, and so was reluctant to go into nursing. Out of curiosity though and following a discussion with my mother, I found out about mental health nursing, and applied. The more I found out about it, and the more clinical experience I gained, the more I felt at home in this line of work.

Society

Often mental health is the subject of stigma, discrimination, labelling and fear. A large amount of work has been undertaken to promote public awareness of mental health by influential organisations such as MIND and Young Minds, and there is a wide-ranging strategy (Health Education England, 2017). Yet crucial to the greater acceptance of the importance of mental health is a change in social attitudes which are often deep rooted. In order to learn, as we identified earlier, it is necessary to appeal to what people already know, and for this information to make sense in the context of their previous experience (Knowles 1980; Knowles et al. 2005). The current thrust of policy in the UK is aimed at promoting mental health and wellbeing. Through people being more willing to talk about how they feel this may in turn make them less prone to experiencing mental ill health to begin with. Yet while promoting psychological wellbeing, this does little to address the specific needs of people with enduring or prolonged mental ill health. Paul Farmer, Chief Executive of MIND has said:

We hear every day from people with mental health problems who tell us that support is getting harder and harder to access as services shrink while demand escalates. Poor mental health can ruin lives, destroy relationships, take away people's independence and can lead to some taking their own lives.

(MIND 2015)

At the same time there is a risk that public perceptions of the considerable distress caused by mental ill health might be reduced.

Activity 10.9

Consider what a person with schizophrenia might look like in terms of physical characteristics and appearance.

- Did they have a specific gender?
- What physical characteristics did they have?
- What does this demonstrate to you about your perceptions of mental health?

Author's own experience

When growing up, my knowledge of mental health nursing was limited to my uncle and cousin. In his late thirties my uncle began to experience schizophrenia-like symptoms. This did not fit the symptomatic profile, as typically schizophrenia has an onset in late adolescence, or early adulthood, yet this was his diagnosis. Also, around that time his son, my cousin, began behaving bizarrely, and also required treatment. Both were inpatients at different times and came back as changed people; they were never the same again, and experienced recurrent relapses. My parents had no idea about the treatment that had been given but acted differently towards my uncle and cousin, distancing themselves to the point of not inviting them into the house should they call round. In hindsight, I realise that this was a result of stigma and fear. I was fascinated as on the one hand the mental health services were secretive and mysterious, yet at the same time seemed to have complete power over people's lives while the treatments provided seemed to be of doubtful efficacy. In recent years I have had further encounters with the mental health services as a member of the public. In spite of my knowledge of the service and the long time since I last encountered the mental health services, a lot was still the same. There is still a sense of mystery and a potent aura of power and control over people's lives. Yet at the same time there is a disappointing sense that care and treatment can at best offer only partial and incomplete solutions. This is perhaps unsurprising, as mental ill health produces such a dramatic and multi-faceted impact on the life of the person and also all of those around them that not everything can be resolved. However, on reflection this experience has led me to be aware of the necessity to remember how individual these experiences are for those affected and for carers, significant others and the person's wider circle.

In this chapter, we have looked at a range of factors that contribute to the establishment of your identity as a qualified nurse. We have different priorities and values as people, and so these will differ between individuals. Looking at ourselves as who we are as individual people as opposed to our identity as nurses will help. The process of learning as a nurse is a matter of seeking to become more human. Increasingly the pre-registration nurse training curriculum is competence led, which may be seen as standardising nursing. Instead and in contrast to this notion, being able to embrace the difference in situations will achieve technical competence and skill. Nursing is about being human and our emotions and feelings resembling and being synchronised to those of our patients and service users.

I hope you have enjoyed this book and find the ideas and concepts to have some value for you in your developing career and life, and wish you enjoyment and satisfaction throughout your nursing career. You are your own best teacher but in order to learn we need to have our eyes and ears open to understand the experiences in which we are involved. Self-compassion, role modelling for junior staff and being aware of your own and others' fitness to practice will stand you in good stead and mean that you experience positive growth but also perform a useful role in the development of your other colleagues as well.

REFERENCES

Allport, G.W. and Odbert, H.S. (1936). Trait names: a psycho-lexical study. *Psychological Monographs*, 47.

Bar-On, R. (2002). Emotional Quotient Inventory: Short (Bar-On EQ-i:S): Technical Manual. Multi-Health Systems, Canada.

Bar-On, R. (2006). The Bar-On model of emotional-social intelligence (ESI). *Psicothema*, 18 (Suppl.): 13–25.

Bowlby, E.J.M. (1997). *Attachment and Loss*, vol. 1: *Attachment*. London: Random House.

Bowlby, E.J.M. (1998a). *Attachment and Loss*, vol. 2: *Separation: Anxiety and Anger*. London: Random House.

Bowlby, E.J.M. (1998b). *Attachment and Loss*, vol. 3: *Loss*. London: Random House.

Brown, C.B. and Lowis, M.J. (2003). Psychosocial development in the elderly: an investigation into Erikson's ninth stage. *Journal of Aging Studies*, 17(4): 415–26.

Carragher, J. and Gormley, K. (2017). Leadership and emotional intelligence in nursing and midwifery education and practice: a discussion paper. *Journal of Advanced Nursing*, 73(1): 85–96.

Cattell, R.B. (1943). The description of personality: basic traits resolved into clusters. *Journal of Abnormal and Social Psychology*, 38: 476–506.

Celikel, F.C. (2011). Personality traits: reflections in the brain. In M.E. Jordan (ed.), *Personality Traits: Theory, Testing and Influences*. New York: Nova Publishers, pp. 161–73.

Clance, P.R. and Imes, S.A. (1978). The imposter phenomenon in high achieving women: dynamics and therapeutic intervention. *Psychotherapy: Theory, Research & Practice*, 15(3): 241–7.

Cloninger, C.R., Przybeck, T.R., Svrakic, D.M. and Wetzel, R. (1994). *The Temperament and Character Inventory (TCI): A Guide to Its Development and Use*. St. Louis: Washington University School of Medicine, Department of Psychiatry.

Delgado, C., Upton, D., Ranse, K., Furness, T. and Foster, K. (2017). Nurses' resilience and the emotional labour of nursing work: an integrative review of empirical literature. *International Journal of Nursing Studies*, 70: 71–88.

Department of Health (DoH) (1999). *Making a Difference: Strengthening the Nursing, Midwifery and Health Visiting Contribution to Health and Healthcare*. https://webarchive. nationalarchives.gov.uk/20120524072447/http://www.dh.gov.uk/prod_consum_dh/ groups/dh_digitalassets/@dh/@en/documents/digitalasset/dh_4074704.pdf, accessed 12 April 2019.

Einstein, A. (n.d.). www.thymindoman.com/einsteins-misquote-on-the-illusion-of-feeling- separate-from-the-whole, accessed 29 August 2019.

Erikson, E. (1968). *Identity, Youth and Crisis*. New York: W.W. Norton.

Erikson, E. (1998). *The Life Cycle Completed*. Extended version with new chapters on the ninth stage by Joan M. Erikson. New York: W.W. Norton.

Fiske, D.W. (1949). Consistency of the factorial structures of personality ratings from different sources. *Journal of Abnormal and Social Psychology*, 44: 329–44.

Greenberger, D., & Padesky, C. A. (1995). *Mind over mood: A cognitive therapy treat- ment manual for clients*. New York, NY, US: Guilford Press.

Goleman, D. (1995). *Emotional Intelligence: Why it Can Matter More than IQ*. New York: Bantam Books.

Goleman, D. (1998). *Working with Emotional Intelligence*. New York: Bantam Books.

Hakamata, Y. and Inada, T. (2011). Structural and functional neuroimaging studies of the anxiety-related personality trait: implications for the neurobiological basis of human anxious personality. In M.E. Jordan (ed.), *Personality Traits: Theory, Testing and Influences*. New York: Nova Publishers, pp. 103–31.

Health Education England (2017). *Action Plan for Mental Health Promotion and Prevention Courses 2016–2020*. www.hee.nhs.uk/sites/default/files/documents/ Action%20plan%20for%20mental%20health%20promotion%20and%20prevention% 20courses%202016-2020.pdf, accessed 4 November 2018.

Heidegger, M. (2003). *Being and Time*, trans. J. Macquarrie and E. Robinson. Oxford: Blackwell Publishing.

Hochschild, A.R. (1983). *The Managed Heart: Commercialization of Human Feeling*. Berkeley: University of California.

Hochschild, A.R. (2003). *The Managed Heart: Commercialization of Human Feeling*. Twentieth anniversary ed. Berkeley: University of California.

Johnson, C.L. and Barer, M. (1993). Coping and a sense of control among the oldest old: an exploratory analysis. *Journal of Aging* 7(1) 67–80.

Knowles, M.S. (1980). *The Modern Practice of Adult Education: Andragogy versus Pedagogy*. Englewood Cliffs, NJ: Prentice Hall.

Knowles, M.S., Holton, E.F. and Swanson, R.A. (2005). *Andragogy in Action: Applying Modern Principles of Adult Education*, 6th ed. London: Elsevier.

Levett-Jones, T. and Lathlean, J. (2008). Belongingness: a prerequisite for nursing students' clinical learning. *Nurse Education in Practice*, 8: 103–11.

Marmot, M. (2010). *Fair Society, Healthy Lives: The Marmot Review – Strategic Review of Health Inequalities in England Post-2010*. www.parliament.uk/documents/fair-society-healthy-lives-full-report.pdf, accessed 30 October 2019.

Mayer, J.D., Salovey, P. and Caruso, D.R. (2004). Emotional intelligence: theory, findings and implications. *Psychological Inquiry*, 15(5): 197–215.

MIND (2015). *Mind Response to King's Fund Briefing on Mental Health Services*. www.mind.org.uk/news-campaigns/news/mind-response-to-kings-fund-briefing-on-mental-health-services/#.W97Kbkx2s2w, accessed 4 November 2018.

Peternelli-Taylor, C. (2011). Is impostor syndrome getting in the way of writing for the *Journal of Forensic Nursing? Journal of Forensic Nursing*, 7: 57–9.

Piaget, J. (2000). *Psychology of the Child*. New York: Basic Books.

Rotter, J. (1966). Generalized expectancies for internal versus external control of reinforcement. *Psychological Monographs*, 80(1): 1–28.

Schouten, J.W. (1991). Selves in transition: symbolic consumption in personal rites of passage and identity reconstruction. *Journal of Consumer Research*, 17(4): 412–25.

Skinner, V. and Wrycraft, N. (2014). *CBT Fundamentals: Theory and Cases*. Maidenhead: McGraw-Hill/Open University.

Svrakic, D.M., Draganic, S., Hill, K., Bayon, C., Przybeck, T.R. and Cloninger, C.R. (2002). Temperament, character and personality disorders: etiologic, diagnostic, treatment issues. *Acta Psychiatrica Scandinavica*, 106: 189–195.

Veazey Brooks, J. and Bosk, C.L. (2012). Remaking surgical socialization: work hour restrictions, rites of passage and occupational identity. *Social Science and Medicine*, 75: 1625–32.

Walker, S., Dwyer, T., Broadbent, M., Moxham, L., Sander, T. and Edwards, K. (2014). Constructing a nursing identity within the clinical environment: the student nurse experience. *Contemporary Nurse*, 49: 103–12.

Whittle, S., Allen, N.B., Lubman, D.I. and Yucel, M. (2006). The neurobiological basis of temperament: towards a better understanding of psychopathology. *Neuroscience and Biobehavioural Reviews*, 30: 511–25.

Index